D1744643

Running For Life

Running For Life

THE ODYSSEY OF A HEART-ATTACK VICTIM'S JOGGING BACK TO HEALTH

by TEX MAULE

Pelham Books - London

First published in Great Britain by PELHAM BOOKS LIMITED
52 Bedford Square, London, W.C.1
1973

© 1972 by Tex Maule

All Rights Reserved. No part of this publication
may be reproduced, stored in a retrieval system,
or transmitted, in any form or by any means,
electronic, mechanical, photocopying, recording
or otherwise, without the prior permission
of the Copyright owner

ISBN 0 7207 0689 0

Printed in Great Britain by
Redwood Press Limited, Trowbridge, Wiltshire
and bound by James Burn at Esher, Surrey

In Memory of My Son

Running For Life

Chapter One /

On Monday morning, March 21, 1966, two days after my fifty-first birthday, I had a massive heart attack.

I didn't know what it was at first. I was drinking coffee with my wife, Dorothy, in the dining area of our Manhattan apartment when I broke out in a cold sweat and felt so nauseated that I could not finish the coffee.

My wife was upset, but I was not seriously worried. I had been up until four in the morning and it was just 8 A.M., so I thought the nausea and the cold sweat were the natural result of a long night of hard work, heavy drinking, chain smoking, tension, and very little sleep. After a few minutes, I felt better and I dressed and packed, preparing to catch a plane to Canada, where I was to cover the Muhammad Ali–George Chuvalo heavyweight championship fight for *Sports Illustrated*, the magazine I work for.

I still felt weak and a little shaky and Dorothy suggested that I postpone the trip for a day but I told her that I was feeling much better and that I would be all right. I hadn't missed a day's work for illness in over ten years.

I had reached the door and was just turning to say good-bye when I broke out in a cold sweat again; the nausea came back so strongly that I had to clench my teeth to keep from vomiting. My legs felt weak and trembly and I put down the bag and leaned against the door for a moment to keep from falling.

"You look terrible," Dorothy said. "What's the matter?"

"I'll be all right in a minute," I said. "I'll sit down until this goes away. I'm just tired."

I walked back in the living room and sat down on the couch and she sat by me, watching me anxiously. I smiled at her and tried to light a cigarette, but my hands were shaking so badly that it seemed to me a long time before I got it lit. I still had had no pain of any kind and, since I had never had any trouble with my heart, I was sure this was only a hangover of some kind. I have never had a hangover in my life, so I didn't know what one felt like.

The cigarette tasted like burning sulphur and made my nausea worse, so I put it out and took three or four deep breaths, which made me feel a little better. My face was wet with sweat and I could feel sweat trickling down my sides, so I stood up and took off my topcoat.

"I think you should go back to bed," Dorothy said.

"If I don't feel better in a few minutes, I will."

I sat still, breathing deeply, and the sweat dried stickily on my face and the nausea began to die down. After five minutes, over Dorothy's strong objection, I got up and started for the door again.

I had taken only five or six steps when the pain in my chest started. It wasn't severe at first, more of a dull growing ache than a pain, but the nausea and the weakness came with it and I went back to the couch and sat down again.

The pain grew and grew, stretching across my chest from arm pit to arm pit. By now it was a crushing pain, as though my chest were being squeezed down by a giant kneeling on me, growing heavier and heavier. It made breathing difficult so that I could no longer take the deep breaths which had relieved me earlier. I was panting with the quick, shallow breaths of a tired puppy and for the first time I thought I was having a heart attack.

Dorothy was crying and I told her it would be all right and sat carefully still, hoping the pain and the pressure would go away. From some medical article I had read a long time ago, I suddenly remembered that if you are having a heart attack, your fingernails turn from pink to blue, and I held up my hand and looked at my fingertips. The nails were bluish.

I stood up gently and began to walk toward the bedroom and said, "Honey, I think you better call Jerry."

I was lucky. Jerry is our family doctor who is also a heart specialist. His office is only twenty minutes from our apartment, and he was in.

I took off my suit coat and lay down on the bed and Dorothy got through to Jerry immediately. He said he would come at once. The nausea returned a hundred times worse and I wasn't strong enough to get up and go to the bathroom, so I rolled off the bed, landing on the floor on my hands and knees and began to vomit. My wife brought something and I retched and vomited for what seemed to me a long time, then she helped me back into the bed.

The pain was still there and the sense of pressure, but the nausea was gone for the moment and I felt a little better and I began trying to convince myself that it was only indigestion, after all.

Jerry must have set some kind of record driving the twenty-odd blocks from his office to our apartment house.

He is a short, rather round man with a cheerful face and an air of implacable good cheer. By the time he came into the bedroom, my daughter, Freddie, who was then eighteen, was up and she and my wife were doing their best to help me and growing more and more frightened. Strangely enough, I never felt afraid; I think I felt more irritated with myself than anything else and apprehensive about not being able to make the trip to cover the fight.

Jerry felt my pulse, listened to my chest, took my blood pressure and an electrocardiogram, and gave me a shot, all in a very few minutes. He never once told me that I had had a heart attack, but early on, I suppose to quiet Dorothy and Freddie and give them something to do as much as for any other reason, he told Dorothy to call the Flower & Fifth Avenue Hospital and get me a room at once and gave Freddie the job of calling an ambulance.

I began to feel embarrassed at being so much trouble and, half an hour later, when the ambulance attendants came into the room with a stretcher, I tried to get up and into it myself. I realized for the first time how serious the situation was when Jerry stopped me.

"Don't move," he said. "Don't even lift your hand. Lie as still as you can. They will do all the work."

The attendants had brought a portable oxygen bottle and mask and Jerry fitted the mask to my face. I breathed oxygen for a long time from that moment on.

Jerry had loosened my shirt and trousers and, once I had been loaded onto the rolling stretcher, he tucked a blanket around me. I felt relieved when he did; I knew we would be going down in the elevator from the eleventh floor and I was not anxious for my neighbors to see me half undressed. Like most New Yorkers, I know none of my neighbors well, but it is undignified enough to be hauled out of your apartment in a stretcher without being exposed as well.

We ran into a small problem getting on the elevator. I suppose when the builders of the apartment house in which I live—a twenty-story affair on the East Side of Manhattan which was put up only about five or six years before my attack—never thought any of the approximately 320 apartment dwellers would ever have to be taken out on a stretcher. The elevators are not wide enough or long enough to take a stretcher.

The attendants solved that by folding the stretcher in the middle, where it is hinged, and I rode down the eleven flights in what I suppose could best be described as a supine crouching position, bent slightly at the waist and knees. The elevator operator, an old friend of mine, looked at me sadly and seemed on the point of saying something, but I think he was, like most people, intimidated by serious, sudden illness. I smiled at him as if to reassure him that it wasn't really as bad as it looked, but I couldn't think of anything to say. I don't think it would have helped much to say, "It's just a small heart attack."

They loaded me into the back of the ambulance, to the deep interest of the doormen and a couple of tenants who happened to be leaving at the same time, and we left for the hospital with the siren going. The shots Jerry had given me earlier had taken effect and I was breathing easier and the pain in my chest had died down until it was only a reminder of what it had been. I remember it was a sparklingly bright, sunshiny day, the kind you get in Manhattan in the early spring about one day in twenty. My wife and daughter were sitting by me in the back of the ambulance and I told them, inanely, that everything would be fine. I don't think I convinced either of them.

Since then, I have tried to remember what I thought about on that trip, but I'm not really very clear. I felt sorry for Dorothy and Freddie, in a detached way, but the sedation Jerry gave me acted much like one of the drugs they administer to make you happy.

I remember I looked out of the window as we went through the crowded early-morning streets of upper Manhattan and saw the healthy people on their way to work—or wherever they were going—and felt no deep sense of sorrow or envy. I suppose if I had not been under sedation, I might have felt fear and sorrow for myself, or more sorrow for Dorothy and my daughter, but all I can clearly remember feeling was that if I was going to die (and I was no more convinced of that than anyone is ever convinced that he is going to die) at least I had died a long way down the road.

I was fifty-one years old and I had done a lot of things in the fifty-one years. I tried, drowsily, to think of all the things I had done and none of them came back to me very clearly, but all of them seemed good—at least in retrospect as the ambulance made its way up Park Avenue on a bright March morning.

I even congratulated myself on not feeling fear, although I didn't deserve nearly as much credit for that as did Jerry and his injections. Unfortunately, Dorothy and Freddie had not had the injections. They felt, in full measure, all the fear and sorrow for me that I could not feel for myself.

Of course, what I did not realize at that time, what I did not realize until quite a long time later, was that I had already begun to retreat into the cocoon that the seriously ill make for themselves. Whether I knew it consciously or not, I had begun to divorce myself a little from the living and their concerns and concentrate upon my own needs, and my first need then and for the next few weeks was to prepare myself for dying by making it easier to leave life.

For me, that need was fulfilled by thinking, however spuriously, that I had gotten a full measure of pleasure out of life and that, if I died, I would not be leaving behind great deeds undone, great books not written, great loves not consummated. I had had a long, very happy time with my wife, I had seen my daughter grow from a lovely child to a lovely young woman. In short I had enjoyed myself.

True, I had not written any great books or done any great deeds, but the books I had written had been good enough in their context and if the deeds had not been great, they had been satisfying. At the time, that seemed enough.

It was a long ride for Dorothy and Freddie with me in the ambulance. Neither of them had left me from the time they knew it was a heart attack, except to make the calls Jerry had asked them to—the calls to the hospital and the ambulance.

"I was afraid, of course," my wife told me later. "But I thought that if I left you, I would be taking away a strength you needed to survive. I thought that as long as I was close to you, I could lend you some of my strength and that you would live."

She does not remember what she thought about in the ambulance and the only thing that my daughter remembers about what must have been a nightmarish trip for both of them was that once I said to her, "Don't be afraid."

One other thing Dorothy remembers is that the ambulance almost stalled climbing a small hill a block or two from the apartment and she thought to herself, "This is all we need!"

My memory of my arrival at the hospital at about 9 A.M. is very vague, since by now the drugs had taken over and I was only hazily aware of what was going on. I remember what seemed a long wait for an elevator; my wife told me later that one elevator was out of order and we had to go to another one. At the second elevator, there was another delay and an old man, sick, was waiting with his wife, and Dorothy, who was on the edge of hysteria, looked at them and said to our daughter, "It doesn't matter for them. They are old."

I was supposed to have a private room, but instead I was put in a room with another patient, again an old man. This must have been morning visiting hours, because his wife was with him.

After a nurse had arranged my oxygen tent—a clear plastic tent which covers the whole bed and, in time, becomes as comforting for a heart patient as the womb must be for a fetus—I was left alone with my wife and daughter and the sick old man and his wife. So I began to vomit again.

My wife and daughter rushed out into the hall for help and the old man left his bed to come to my aid. This is something else you learn very quickly in a hospital—the patients, by and large, are much more sympathetic and thoughtful and will go to greater lengths to help you than the hospital personnel.

I don't know what was wrong with the sick old man. I never learned his name, because I was put in a private room not long after that, but one of the things that comes back to me through the haze of drugs was his anxious, kind face and the voice of his wife.

"Papa, papa!" she cried. "Get back into bed! They'll take care of him."

Ten or fifteen minutes later a nurse and two interns arrived and made repairs on me and the oxygen tent, which they discovered had not been functioning before. My wife was crying in the hall and Jerry was parking his car and, as well as I can remember, I was watching pro-

)11(

ceedings with a rather pleasant sense of detachment, even while I vomited.

When I had been taken care of, my wife came back into the room and the ambulance driver, who had been waiting in the wings, presented her with the bill from Keefe and Keefe ambulance service. He wouldn't leave until she had given him a check.

By now, Jerry had come back and he arranged for a private room for me and I was moved. The private room may have been an improvement, but I couldn't tell by then. The first time I was aware of it was a long time later, after I had made an extended visit to intensive care. When I came back to my room ten days later, I was impressed by the pile of bird droppings on the window sill. I could have made a fortune if I had been a guano dealer and had had the energy to reap that crop.

My memories of the days I spent in the private room before I was taken to the intensive care section are blurred, since I was under constant sedation. I was moved into the private room Monday afternoon; I needed twenty-four-hour nursing care and my wife spent a good deal of the time with a friend of hers trying to locate the necessary nurses, which is not as easy as it sounds.

She asked me several times if I wanted her to call the office and tell them that I was sick, but I asked her not to, since I felt that I might recover in a few hours and go on to cover the fight in Canada. She called the office in the early afternoon when it became very clear that I wouldn't be going anywhere for a long time.

At one point, Jerry took her aside and explained to her exactly what had happened to me and drew a diagram of the heart, showing her how much damage had been done by the occlusion.

"Tex has had a massive heart attack," he said. "But he's lucky about one thing. He hasn't gone into heart failure."

Once I had reached the hospital, the immediate danger was over. Many victims of a heart attack die simply because they are not in an area where they can be quickly treated, and the damaged heart, with no help, dies. I was lucky in reaching the hospital within an hour after the attack.

My daughter was a student at Bard College and she left to go back to school in the early afternoon. Although I was sedated and sleepy, I agreed with her mother that it would be better for her to return to school, since there was little she could do and the crisis had passed. She left very reluctantly.

Dorothy finally located a male practical nurse to sit with me and he reported for duty at noon and promptly gave me a bath, which is one thing which is never done to a man who has just suffered a heart attack.

Luckily, I survived the rigors of the bath and that particular nurse never returned to duty after Jerry learned what he had done. When Dorothy eventually hired three nurses to keep constant watch over me, she still remained in the visitors' room of the hospital herself for three days and nights. As the nurses finished their shifts, they would report to her to collect for the day's work.

From Monday to Wednesday, I improved steadily. I was being fed intravenously and I was attached to an electronic electrocardiograph machine, which monitored my heartbeat constantly. Although I spent all my time on my back in my oxygen tent, I was getting better.

During the time I was punchy from the drugs, I have a faint memory of thinking of brilliant plots for novels and short stories and making a strong effort to record them mentally so that I could write them when I recovered. I haven't any recollection of them now.

Dorothy tells me that during this time I made motions as though I were turning the pages of a book or writing, and one of the nurses told her that this was not unusual.

"They do what they do for a living," she said. "He's writing."

I was supposed to be constantly under the eye of a nurse during this critical period and Dorothy, sitting endless hours in the visitors' room near my room, told the nurses that if they wanted a coffee break or to leave the room for any other reason she would be glad to sit in for them while they were gone.

By Wednesday, I was well enough so that I no longer needed heavy sedation and Dorothy fed me the first food I had taken by mouth since the attack, a bowl of Jello. I was well enough to want to read and the nurse said that it would be better to let me read than argue with me about it.

I don't remember the name of the book I read, but I do remember being surprised at how heavy it was and how tired it made me to turn the pages. That was the first time I realized how weak I was.

Still, by Wednesday evening the picture was much brighter. I had survived the first shock of the attack and rallied and the prognosis was certainly getting better day by day, as my heart recovered from the damage done to it.

I was well enough by Wednesday evening that Dorothy, who had not left the hospital, was persuaded to go home that night and get some sleep. She was preparing to leave around 11:30 P.M. when an intern told her that I had had a setback and was in heart failure. He said I might be dying.

I indeed had a setback, but not from natural causes; the nurse on duty had left me to go for coffee or to the bathroom, without calling Dorothy to watch me for her.

I should explain here that the bedpan is, quite possibly, the most totally useless device ever invented for a man who is so sick that he must lie flat on his back in bed. It requires far more exertion to hoist yourself onto the damned thing than it would if an orderly helped the nurse sit you on a portable potty. The combination of my inability to use the bedpan and reluctance to try it in front of the nurses had reduced me to a state of near eruption.

When I saw the nurse leave the room, I decided that I would get out of bed (since I was under only light sedation) take the four or five steps across the room to the bathroom, and be back in bed before she knew I had left.

I detached myself from the tube being used for intravenous feeding, from another tube which allowed a drug designed to maintain my blood pressure seep into me, and from the leads which attached me to the electrocardiograph machine. Then I lifted the oxygen tent aside and climbed over the low rail at the side of the bed.

I could barely stand, but I tried to walk across the room. I staggered a few steps, then fell forward into the bathroom, hitting my forehead on the edge of the lavatory and inflicting a deep, inch-long cut just between and about an inch above my eyebrows.

I remember feeling shock and surprise at the blood that spurted out and covered my face and hands. And I remember climbing painfully to my feet again, but there was no pain from the cut on my head. When I got up, I staggered backward a step or two, then fell again and hit the back of my head on one of the big, heavy metal oxygen tanks next to my bed.

I must have either knocked myself out or passed out then, because the next thing I remember, I was up again, being held by an orderly and a nurse. The room seemed crowded and I struggled feebly trying to get away. At that time, what I wanted most to do was to go home.

By the time Dorothy had been brought to the room by the intern, the gash in my head had been bandaged and I was back in bed under the oxygen tent, plucking aimlessly at the air as if I were trying to catch butterflies.

I suppose I had been given more sedation, because, although I remember Dorothy coming in, I don't remember talking to her. I must have been quite a sight. She told me later that my face was chalk white, so that the bloodstains stood out like the red lettering on a "Danger!" sign.

I was raving, out of my mind, but I recognized her.

"Pack the books," I said. "We're going home."

She broke into tears and turned away. As she walked out of the room crying I said, "How come you're walking so funny?"

The rest of that night I know of only by hearsay, since I was unconscious, and only a shaky heartbeat or two away from death.

Dorothy became hysterical and called Jerry, who lives in Scarsdale, and told him that they were killing her husband and he told her to calm down.

"What's your version of the story?" he asked her. He knew roughly what had happened since an intern had called him earlier. When Dorothy had told him, he advised her to go home and calm down, neither of which she did.

She sat in the visitors' room and watched the scurrying in and out of my room. The nurse who had walked away and left me unattended came to collect her twenty-eight dollars for the shift.

Crying hopelessly, Dorothy told her, "You killed my husband! You don't deserve any money! Why didn't you call me?"

"I was only gone ten minutes," the woman said sullenly.

For some reason, Dorothy gave her the check, and when it was safely in hand, the nurse turned to a friend who had come in with her.

"That's how they show their appreciation," she said.

At 2:30 A.M. my wife called my brothers, who live in Texas. They are my half brothers; their last name is Wilson and she had not told them I was sick before, not wanting to worry them. Both of them are younger than I; Pat is a doctor and Bubba a real estate dealer. They arrived about noon Thursday.

I was in heart failure, my heart too weak to pump enough blood to sustain life for long, and Jerry and the hospital staff were having a difficult time maintaining my blood pressure. Jerry, in tears, told Dorothy that it looked very bad.

Dorothy was in the hall outside the elevators, surrounded by three close friends and her mother, talking to Jerry, when the elevator doors opened and my brothers came out.

"It was like in the old Western movies, when the Indians are about to wipe out the wagon train and the cavalry arrives," Dorothy told me later. "I don't know why, but when those two stocky Texans came, I felt saved. My friends were all women. I didn't have a man to lean on and now I had two. And I couldn't have asked for two better ones."

Despite the fact that I was in heart failure, with my life flickering from minute to minute, I had not been transferred to intensive care. I was still in the private room.

Late in the afternoon, I was transferred to intensive care. Pat, my brother who is the doctor, asked if the hospital had an intensive care unit, then suggested to Jerry that I should be transferred there.

Dorothy found out I was going to be transferred when a nurse from the unit came down and told her that they were going to do the best they could to save my life, but that they had very strict rules. She would be allowed to visit me only for five minutes, twice a day. She seemed to Dorothy a forbidding and stern woman, but she was much more relaxed once I had been admitted.

I don't remember the transfer, but two things, medically, saved my life. One was the arrival of my brother Pat and the other was the transfer, at his behest, to intensive care.

Chapter Two /

I was lucky to survive the three days in the hospital before I got to intensive care; once there, I was home free. The nurses and the rest of the personnel in intensive care were as good as the private nurse who had almost let me die was bad.

Intensive care is precisely what the name says. Once you are admitted to an intensive care ward, your every moment is monitored by people or machines and the people care about what happens to you. They do not have too many patients to care for, obviously, since every one of their patients requires the utmost in help simply to survive.

For hours on end before I went into intensive care, my brother, with Jerry's approval, had sat by my bed regulating my intake of the blood-pressure drug minute by minute, trying to nurse my failing heart into providing enough blood pressure to keep the other vital organs active. This is a delicate, difficult thing; later he told me that he did not think he could take the responsibility of controlling my life and death for so long. But he did, magnificently.

Thursday night, finally, after I had been admitted to the special unit and there was nothing else my brother or anyone else could do for me, Dorothy, my brothers, her friend Sharon (who, with Marion, another friend, had spent hours at the hospital with her) all went home and relaxed. They got drunk and they damn well earned the right. I don't know what I did, but whatever the healthy people in the intensive care unit did, they did right. I was still alive on Friday, with brighter prospects of continuing to live.

Friday afternoon, Freddie returned from Bard and came in to see me. She was allowed only a few minutes and I spent most of the time complaining to her that an intern had taken thirteen stabs at finding a vein through which I could be fed. This was true, but it was not the fault of the intern. My veins, pumped into only very feebly by my heart, were hard to find and harder to hold still.

When Freddie went back out to see her mother, she was destroyed. She had felt guilty about leaving me on Monday when the heart attack occurred; the change in my physical appearance from Monday to Friday was profound.

Jerry explained it to her rather well.

"When you left him Monday," he said, "you left a

healthy man who had had a heart attack. When you saw him today, you saw a man who was sick with heart disease and has been for five days."

I was twenty pounds lighter by then and the only solid food I had had in five days was the bowl of Jello my wife had fed me just before my aborted trip to the john. My heart was recovering, but very, very slowly. I was wired to a continuous EKG machine, which showed my heartbeat as a bouncing, bright light on a television screen and I had tubes in me for a variety of reasons, none of them comfortable. I must have looked like a death's head, but, as I grew more and more aware of my surroundings, I wasn't unhappy.

The intensive care unit is a ward, so that I had neighbors to watch and speculate about. Unfortunately, during the time I was there, two of them died, but they had come in as even more forlorn cases than I and no one really expected them to live. I don't recall what their ailments were; both were postoperative patients and they didn't last long enough to make a clear impression.

I do remember a stick-thin, gray man with a nose like a beak and a large, devoted Italian family, which took turns sitting around his bed during the brief visiting periods and weeping silently. I don't know what he had but one of the first things I noticed, when I came far enough out of sedation and far enough from the shadow of my own imminent death to look around me, was his breathing.

Each tortured, rattling gasp of breath was, I thought, his last. I first became aware of it in the early hours of the morning, when the ward was quiet, dimly lit; the face of my personal TV program, recording the tribulations of my heart, was the brightest point in my night-life.

I woke up to a slow, measured "Haaaauuugh!" This was followed by a gurgle, a silence, and the same sound repeated. From inside the oxygen tent, the sound was muted, but it had all the finality of a death rattle. I tried to locate the source, but I couldn't and I dropped off to sleep, the easy drowsiness of a sick man. It's a sleep which is a refuge, and if you're sick enough you slip into it gratefully. If you're too sick, you're afraid to go to sleep; I saw patients fight drugs and sleepiness and shake their heads to stay awake and I'm sure it was because awake they knew they were still alive. Only a couple of times did I feel afraid to go to sleep; most of the time I had a strong feeling that I would live. The times when that feeling would have been an off-the-book bet, I was too drugged to know what was going on. You have to have some luck, some times.

The old man lived on precariously for a few days then, miraculously, began slowly to grow better. When he was taken out of intensive care and returned to a ward, breathing easily and gaining weight, his face pink instead of gray, I felt as if I had won a personal victory. Surely if he had survived, my own case was not too critical.

I stayed in intensive care for ten days. When I first went in, I was under heavy sedation and not rational, so that Dorothy was afraid for a while that my brain had been damaged during the time I was in heart failure.

An intern told her that I had no mental damage and proved it.

"What's your favorite football team?" he asked me.

"The Green Bay Packers," I said fuzzily.

"Who is their coach?"

"Vince Lombardi."

The nursing care in the special unit was as good as nursing can be. The girls on each shift were gentle, intelligent, and extraordinarily competent and the residents and interns were good as well. All of them were expert in taking care of heart patients.

Any victim of a heart attack is very fortunate if he is taken to a hospital that has an intensive care unit like this one. The mortality rate for patients under ordinary hospital routine is significantly higher than it is for patients in intensive care. The slightest variation in heart rate, blood pressure, respiration, or any other physical condition is noted immediately and medical help is instantaneous. I am sure that I would not have survived the fall and subsequent heart failure had the hospital not had this unit; of course, I would not have had either if the nursing care in the private room had been remotely adequate.

I had a private nurse for the dog watch (from midnight to morning) in intensive care, a man who had worked for the Joseph Kennedy family. Soon after I had been admitted, my wife was called at midnight and told that another emergency had occurred; my brothers, who had not been to New York before, were touring Greenwich Village and Dorothy left a message for them with her mother and rushed to the hospital.

When she reached the hospital, the emergency was over. I had tried to do the same thing I had done in the private room but this time when I tried to climb out of the bed, the nurse was there, alert, and restrained me. Had I had the same nurse in the private room earlier, I probably would not have been in intensive care at all.

I did no serious damage to myself this time.

For some reason, I still found it very difficult to use a bedpan and eventually I had to be catheterized in order to relieve the pressure on my bladder. It took me a week or ten days before I was able to use the bedpan at all; luckily, I was being fed intravenously much of that time and the problem was not a severe one.

Dorothy had one more shock during this time. The continuous EKG I was connected to constantly was once used briefly to record the heart patterns of a tiny blue baby, a Puerto Rican infant who was to be operated on later. The heart surgeon brought him in and connected him to the EKG recorder, placing his crib immediately next to my bed, then left for a while.

While he was gone, Dorothy came in and stopped short when she saw the baby.

"All the time I thought it was just a heart attack," she said. "What are we going to name it?"

The first food I took by mouth was an eggnog. I hadn't eaten in over a week and I was fairly scrawny as well as dehydrated.

When Jerry suggested the eggnog, I refused it, since I am reluctant to drink eggnog even during the Christmas season. Freddie knew how to get me to try it.

"Put a jigger of scotch in it," she told Jerry.

He did and I took the eggnog and began eating again. The food tasted delicious, which is an indication of just how starved I was. The catering for this hospital is done by Horn & Hardart, not high on any list of gourmet restaurants.

Later Jerry prescribed two ounces of whiskey for me

before dinner every night. I looked forward to the drink each evening, but some of the pleasure of drinking is destroyed when the drink is poured by a nurse who measures it out precisely in a test tube before pouring it into a paper cup. However, it was a lot better than nothing at all.

I was still plugged into the EKG, punctured by various tubes dripping drugs of one kind or another into my veins to bolster my heart, and unable to move much; but I could read light books and the days were not monotonous. I'm not quite sure what kind of shots are necessary to keep a heart patient alive but I do know that there are many of them.

One of the most painful was a shot I was given each night in my hip, first on one side then the other. Most hypodermics have needle-sized points and they sting when you're jabbed but it's nothing to worry about. This one had a point about as big around as a pencil; most of the time when I got hit with it, I felt as though I had been stabbed.

Except for one night, when an Indian intern made the rounds with the resident who usually punctured me.

"How many more of these shots do I have to take?" I asked the resident as I turned carefully on my side and pulled down my pajama pants.

"Not many," he said. "Do they hurt?"

"Damn right."

The Indian, a small, gentle man who had taken his medical degree in India, said, "May I do this one?"

"Sure," the resident said.

I felt his fingers gently probing my upper hip then I felt the needle go in. I had the physical sense of the needle cutting through the flesh, but no pain at all.

"How did you do that?" I asked him when I lay back.

"In my country, we know the areas where there is no pain," he said, and smiled. "I just found one."

"Teach him," I said, nodding at the resident.

I don't think he did. The resident gave me the shot the next evening and it hurt, as usual. I don't know what happened to the Indian intern, but I missed him.

I left intensive care about ten days after I had entered and returned to my private room. When I was wheeled in, I was almost suffocated by the smell of stale flowers; the room was full of flowers that had been sent by friends in the days immediately after my heart attack, put in the room, and left there to wilt. I asked why they had not been distributed to other patients in the wards where they might have been of some use, but no one seemed to know the answer. They were sent to me, this was my room (for which I paid all the time I was in intensive care even though it was not used), and the flowers had to be delivered to that room and stay there.

By the time I came back to the room, most of them had died and had to be thrown away. I can't say that I was upset at the time; the fact that I was being transferred from intensive back to a private room meant that I had improved a great deal and that was all that concerned me at the moment.

The rest of my stay in the hospital was relatively uneventful. The meals did not improve and the service in the private room was not nearly as efficient or as quick as it had been in intensive, but I survived.

In the days and weeks immediately following a coronary, your life is tentative. You are aware of everything that is going on around you and interested, after you have passed the period of heavy sedation and are reasonably conscious again, but one part of your mind is always monitoring your heart, waiting apprehensively for a small pain or a constriction or anything out of the ordinary which would indicate trouble starting up again.

My blood pressure was spectacularly low during the early stages of my attack and it did not come back up to normal for a long time, but my heart seemed to me to be ticking away steadily enough, as far as I could tell from my own continuous mental electrocardiogram. I spent the days reading and the nights watching television and I grew more and more anxious to get home.

I was allowed to sit up in bed for meals, then allowed to get out of bed to go to the bathroom when necessary. I think the latter privilege meant more to me than the first solid food I ate.

I spent three weeks in the hospital room; I might have come home sooner but one night, while I was watching *The Late Show*, I began to feel an ache in my left arm which spread through my chest. I tried to ignore it at first, hoping that it would diminish, but it grew more and more severe and at last I pushed the button to call the night nurse.

When she came, two segments of a Western and three commercials later, I was in deep pain and I told her what had happened. She took my temperature and went off to find an intern or the resident on duty, leaving me lying uncomfortably on my side with the thermometer in a most undignified place, unable to see the TV.

She returned in due time, plucked out the thermometer, read it, and said, "The doctor will be here as soon as he can."

He did come, eventually, and examined me and said that it was nothing serious and gave me something to put me to sleep. I missed the end of the movie.

Again, on a Saturday night when my wife was with me, I had the pain and went through almost the same experience, except that Dorothy insisted on calling Jerry, who was at home in Scarsdale, about to take his wife to dinner, happily. Jerry talked to the resident, who examined me and said I was only having angina pains, the severe chest pains that occur when the heart muscle does not get enough oxygen.

The pain persisted and Jerry finally came in and took an EKG, which confirmed the resident's diagnosis. He gave me some sedation, too, and I missed *The Late Show* again. By this time I had become a real fan of old Western movies.

The angina never recurred after that and I was ready to go home within a few days. This time I went in a cab, going down to the hospital entrance in a wheelchair, pushed by a very kind, gentle Puerto Rican man who had given me a bath every morning. He was a very good nurse and adept at bathing me, even loving. I don't think the fact that he was homosexual had anything to do with his care; certainly I could not have been the object of anyone's affection then.

One morning he asked me, "What do you think about the gay people, Mr. Maule?"

"Right now I have enough problems of my own," I told him. "The gay people don't disturb me. They have their lives to live, too."

"Thank you," he said, rather obscurely.

The cashier at the hospital held up my departure briefly. The total bill came to nearly six thousand dollars, including the time I spent in intensive care and all of the lab work necessary; luckily, I had medical insurance that paid for nearly all of it. But my telephone bill, about sixty dollars, was not included and the bookkeeping department wanted it paid before I was released.

Dorothy wanted to argue, since the telephone had been in the private room and had not been used at all while I was in intensive and only sparingly after that, but I told her to pay it. I wanted to get home.

Chapter Three /

I spent the next three weeks at home in bed, gaining strength very slowly. Some of the time I used to read what I could about the nature of heart disease, so I would have a clear idea of what had happened to me.

I was taking digitoxin and coumadin daily, the digitoxin to regulate my heartbeat and the coumadin to keep my blood thin and thus to lessen the chance of another clot stopping up a coronary artery, with very likely fatal results this time. It was a difficult time for my wife, who had to take over the duties of nurse and put up with my increasing impatience to be up and active.

Eventually I began to walk slowly around the apartment and I remember I felt I had passed a milestone when I was allowed to take a shower by myself. The road back from extensive heart damage is a long, difficult one and I was taking only the first tottering steps. I would probably have been much more despondent had I known just how long a road lay before me at that time.

It was no consolation to find that I was by no means alone in what had happened to me.

Nearly a million Americans die of heart disease every year, I discovered. No other cause of death—disease, automobile accidents, the war in Vietnam—kills anywhere near as many people. The situation is not getting better, either. Although we have finally begun to cut down on the number of auto deaths by improved safety devices in the cars themselves and we are reducing the toll in the Vietnam war by cutting down our commitment, we are losing more and more people to heart disease.

If you are a male, the odds are only four to one against your developing heart disease of one kind or another. Nearly one in three people who die in the United States each year die of coronary arteriosclerosis, better known to the moribund public as hardening of the arteries.

When I had my coronary occlusion—when I had to put down my bag and go back to the couch because of the nausea and the pain in my chest—the odds were only three to two that I would live for another month. The chances were, actually, only four to one that I would live long enough to make it to the hospital, because about 20 percent of the unfortunates who suffer heart attacks die in the first hour. Another 20 percent lasts only a few weeks.

By the time I read this I had, of course, survived those first few weeks, but I found I had no great cause for celebration. Of the victims who survive the early perils and return to a relatively normal life, one in five can expect to die of a second heart attack within five years. Four to one is not a bad price on a horse, but it's a frighteningly bad price on your life—especially when the span is only five years.

Well, as I write this, I have finished the five years and I feel much stronger and healthier than I did in the years just preceding the heart attack. My heart still has scars, but it bangs away.

When the circulation of a coronary artery is stopped by a clot—when an occlusion occurs—the heart, which is a muscle like any other muscle in the body, reacts the way your calf muscle would if you tied a tight tourniquet just below your knee and tried to run. First, it hurts, then the part denied blood quite literally dies.

If the area of the heart affected by the occlusion is big enough, you die too. In my case, there was enough of the heart functioning to keep me alive during the long, slow healing process.

During the six or eight months just preceding my heart attack, I had been exercising for the first time in many years. I was not taking exercise through any fear of a heart attack; indeed, I had no idea at all that I might suffer one. But my belt size was creeping up and I was gaining weight and finding it a bit difficult to bend over and lace my shoes over a belly that had grown to the size of a volleyball and was moving on to basketball proportions.

So I did the Royal Canadian Air Force exercises and watched my diet a bit, although I did not quit drinking or smoking. My weight came down a little and I began to feel more fit, but the most important effect of this pre-heart-attack exercise was that it developed some collateral circulation in my heart.

A working heart, which is regularly given loads above and beyond the normal requirements of daily living, develops additional circulation in the heart muscle itself. It grows stronger and bigger, just as the bicep muscle grows stronger and bigger if you do chins or curls with a bar bell.

I hadn't been taking very much exercise. I spent about fifteen minutes a day four days a week, including two or three minutes of running in place, but I had spent enough time to develop some collateral circulation.

"If your heart hadn't been strengthened by the exercise you took before the heart attack, the attack might have killed you outright," Jerry told me after I had come home. "You had built it up enough so that it could accept the damage done and still function. A weaker heart might have quit completely."

Of course exercise was no concern of mine for a long time after I came out of the hospital. I took my meals in bed for two of the three weeks I was confined, and when I was finally allowed to get out of bed it was for only fairly brief periods. I had to move carefully and slowly so that my damaged heart would not be subject to any sudden strain.

When I started moving about a bit, I was put down again by another ailment, this one not related to the heart disease but to the hours I had spent in bed. One night, after I had spent an hour or two up and around, I awoke with excruciating pain extending from the small of my back down my right leg.

This pain was far more severe than the pain I had

suffered when the heart attack struck. I had all I could do to keep from howling; the slightest movement created a peak of pain in my back and leg that I can describe only as a toothache multiplied by a thousand.

This started at about three o'clock in the morning, an ungodly hour for any ailment to occur since no doctors are readily available. Jerry had been attentive and conscientious in coming back over and over again to see me; it may seem only right that a doctor should visit a patient regularly in his home, but home calls by modern physicians are not that usual.

I took aspirin and tried to keep quiet so that I wouldn't awaken Dorothy, who had had a difficult time acting as a twenty-four-hour nurse with no help. The aspirin didn't even blunt the agony and, finally, remembering dimly that back pain could be alleviated by lying on a hard surface, I lowered myself gingerly from the bed to the floor.

Lying flat on my back on the floor beside the bed, I wondered if this new development had anything to do with my heart. I put my fingertips against the big artery in my neck to check my pulse and it was regular and as strong as it had ever been since the heart attack. I had no pain in my chest, so I decided that this must be something entirely new.

I didn't want to call Jerry if I could help it, but at about five in the morning, I could no longer take the pain. Dorothy was awake by then and I asked her to call him. She woke him up and he came in immediately.

My problem turned out to be one that often affects patients who have spent a long time in bed, then become ambulatory again. I had pinched the sciatic nerve in my back, a massive nerve extending down the leg and it was, indeed, like a king-sized toothache.

"You'll have to take it easy," Jerry said, after he had given me a shot to put me to sleep. "It would probably help to get a bed board to put under the mattress, too."

The pain passed in a few days and I got up again and moved about the apartment creakily, like an old man. Before now I had not had time to think ahead to what my future held. When you are very sick, I believe you spend most of your energy in day-to-day survival, not trying to look too far into a future that is uncertain, at best.

But by the time I had recovered from the sciatica and had begun to look forward to getting out of bed for good, I had to face the fact that I was not the robust, strong man I had always thought myself. Almost all of my life I had been an athlete, stronger than most, almost sinfully free of illness, conscious of the fact that, in most physical confrontations, the odds in my favor would usually be better than even.

During my time in the hospital and at home, I had, for lack of any more exciting thing to do, grown a beard, which I trimmed into a Vandyke. One morning, watching myself in the mirror as I trimmed the beard, I tried to assess the face I was shaving as though it belonged to a stranger, a clearly impossible thing to do.

But I had enough objectivity to understand that it was a face that looked years older than the one I had shaved the morning I prepared to leave for Canada to cover the Ali–Chuvalo fight. There were wrinkles that had not been evident then and it seemed to me my hair had turned whiter. The beard didn't help a hell of a lot.

Unfortunately, it had come in almost pure white.

I was shaving because, for the first time since the heart attack, I was going to go outside under my own power. It was a warm May day in New York, and Jerry had said that I could take a very short walk if I were careful. When you have been confined to home and hospital as long as I had, a short walk outdoors is the equivalent of a vacation in Hawaii.

As a writer for *Sports Illustrated*, I had led an active life, most of it involved with travel, pressure, long irregular hours, tension. I had not asked Jerry about what kind of activity I could try when I was able to go back to work; I had been reluctant to face that particular problem.

I felt strange as I dressed and prepared to go down to the street with Dorothy. It had been a long time since I had prepared to go out; riding down in the elevator, I felt weak and fragile, a feeling I had never had in my life.

Outside our apartment in Manhattan, the street climbs gently to the north, slants down toward the south, where the East River bends in to make it a dead end.

We decided that I would walk up the slight hill first, instead of having to climb after I had walked a couple of blocks and would be, presumably, tired. So very slowly, with Dorothy hovering solicitously at my side, I walked for two blocks up the street, negotiating a curb en route, walked east to a small park overlooking the river, and stood and watched the tugs go by for a while.

I had thought I would feel stronger. I suppose most people have a tendency to overestimate their recuperative ability; certainly I did. My wife and I stood for four or five minutes looking at the river. Then she asked me if we shouldn't start back; I agreed.

I was glad that the two blocks back were downhill. I didn't want to let Dorothy see how tired I was, but I was very happy to go back to bed when we reached the apartment.

In the next few weeks, I took longer and longer walks until I could move with some freedom and without listening anxiously to the thump of my heart. I went back to work a little over two months after the attack, staying in the office only a few hours a day, but I knew that I would have to test myself eventually.

Before the heart attack, I had been scheduled to cover the World Cup soccer championships in London during July; it was now mid-June and I had not yet made a trip or done a story since my return to work.

The American and National football leagues had made peace during my convalescence and my managing editor asked me if I would like to do a story with Tex Schramm, the general manager of the Dallas Texans, on the behind-the-scenes negotiation that had gone on before the merger. It meant a trip to Dallas, but it would not be a difficult story; I had known Schramm for many years, since I had worked for him as publicity director for the Los Angeles Rams in 1951.

I asked Jerry what he thought about it and he said, "You're not an invalid. Take it easy and you'll be all right."

If you have never had a heart attack, it will be difficult for you to understand what happens the first time you venture out into the world completely on your own. No matter how well you feel (and I didn't feel that well) you move apprehensively.

I hadn't been on an airplane since the heart attack and I was not sure how I would feel, at the altitude pre-set for the cabin. It's not high, but it's not sea level, either, and a damaged heart needs all the oxygen it can get. But I remembered that the planes carry oxygen in convenient containers with masks that drop down in case, in the words of the airlines, "cabin pressure should be reduced."

If cabin pressure is reduced, you're in deep trouble, and I thought, as I fastened my seat belt, that under that kind of stress I'd probably have no need for the oxygen anyway. Air emergencies aren't the best thing in the world for post-cardiac patients.

There were no emergencies on the flight to Dallas, but I had a very personal fright of my own. I had not smoked a cigarette since my heart attack and had had very little to drink. The two shots before dinner that Jerry had allowed me in the hospital was all, even after I returned to work.

But I felt pretty good when the flight took off. I had a couple of vodka martinis before lunch, wine with, and a brandy after, and in the euphoria engendered by the proper amount of alcohol, I picked up the little four-cigarette sample pack the airlines used to give you with lunch, before there were health warnings on regular packs.

I looked at the cigarettes a little while, then I thought, well, one won't hurt. Just to see what it tastes like.

So I lit a cigarette and inhaled deeply. For a few seconds I felt the pleasure any smoker would feel, I suppose, after having gone for months without a cigarette. Then I felt sick at the stomach and I broke out in a clammy sweat and, for ten minutes, I thought I was having another heart attack.

I wasn't. The nausea passed and the faint feeling and the cold sweat with it. The stewardess stopped and looked at me with concern and asked, "Are you all right, sir?" and I nodded, but I wasn't sure. A few minutes later, when I had regained my composure, I got up and went to the john and looked at myself. I was still pale and the white beard made me look a hundred years old. I washed my face and held out my hand to look at my fingernails. They weren't blue, but my hand was shaking and I was glad to get back to my seat and rest.

By the time the flight reached Dallas, I had recovered completely. That does not mean that I felt completely healthy. It takes a long time after a heart attack before you feel like that.

There are so many small things that you take for granted with a heart that has never given you trouble. I never checked my bags before the heart attack because I don't like to lose time waiting to claim them, but on this trip I checked my small bag because I didn't want to have the physical exertion of carrying it the half mile or so that you must walk from where a plane parks to where a cab parks.

While I waited for the bag to make its ride on the carrousel so that I could point it out to a redcap, I went to the counter to rent a car. I had never thought about that one way or another before, but now, as I waited for the girl to make out the contract, I thought about it.

This would be the first time I had driven a car since the attack. I had never thought twice about driving a car before; I'm a competent driver and I have driven on the freeways of Los Angeles and the crowded midtown streets of Manhattan with no difficulty.

But now I thought about how I had felt on the plane for ten minutes and I wondered if that were a one-time thing or if it might happen again—while I was driving at sixty miles an hour on the expressway in to my motel. Given recovery time, I could survive. Given an automobile traveling at a speed requiring split-second reactions from the driver, I might kill not only myself, but someone else as well.

The girl gave me the keys and the papers and I had a redcap take my bag out to the car. I took inventory of how I felt as I walked out into the hot late-afternoon sun in Dallas; my legs were a little weak, but I felt clear-headed and well and I felt sure that I would be able to drive well enough.

I stayed in the slow right-hand lane on the expressway and drove slowly, and I made it to the motel easily. I checked in and called Schramm and set up a dinner date with him, then lay down in the air-conditioned cool of the room and closed my eyes.

I must have slept for an hour or two. Another thing I would have to get used to now was the fact that I grew very tired toward late afternoon; sometimes my legs felt like lead and ached and I had to sleep. When I awakened, I still felt tired, but I showered and drove to Schramm's house and we had dinner and talked for a couple of hours about the story.

I had found out when I went back to the office for the first time that you must expect people to look at you appraisingly when you have come off a heart attack.

Schramm concealed his feelings when he met me and said, with the extra emphasis most people use when seeing you after a long illness, that I looked very good. Of course, I did not. I had lost a great deal of weight, I was pale, and I moved with the unconscious super care that most post-cardiac patients use in the first weeks and months after they return to the workaday world.

It becomes something you don't even think about after a while. You don't walk up a flight of stairs briskly; you move step by step, pausing if there is a landing, trying to avoid placing any unnecessary strain on your heart, aware all the time of your breathing and the heart rhythm.

Sitting at a table on the patio near the pool at Schramm's house, I felt well enough, but when my drink was empty, Tex didn't suggest I fix my own, as he would have done three months before. He got up and fixed it himself. It becomes very easy after a little to accept this kind of extra-solicitous attention and to expect it and so you become more and more sedentary, more and more willing to have things done for you rather than to do them yourself.

So you get a bare minimum of exercise, which is what doctors wanted you to have not too long ago. And there are heart ailments still which require your exerting as little physical effort as possible, but mine was not one. My heart was a weakened muscle and a scarred and damaged one, but it needed exercise to maintain its tone, too.

I returned to New York with no more trouble and wrote the story of the merger. This was June and I was due to go to London to cover the World Cup soccer championships the first of July, a much more demanding assignment physically. The soccer matches would be played in London, Liverpool, Everton, Swansea, and other places in Britain, and would require considerable travel over a period of a month.

I was seeing Jerry every week then, for electrocardiograms and for continuing treatment and I asked him if he thought the trip would be dangerous for me.

"No more than staying home," he said. "You'll have to take it easy, but I don't see any reason why you can't go. You'll have to find a physician in London to see every week to check your blood count and regulate the amount of coumadin you take, but other than that, you should be fine."

Coumadin is a blood-thinning drug which helps ensure that no new clot will form and occlude the coronary artery again. The only problem with coumadin is that it must be taken very carefully—too little is useless, too much can cause internal capillary bleeding as the blood seeps out of the small blood vessels. Since the clotting factor of the blood is impaired, the patient becomes, in effect, a bleeder while taking coumadin and must always carry another drug with him in case he cuts himself and cannot stop the bleeding.

I went to London with my wife and spent a month covering the World Cup. During the month, I discovered that I did not have to baby myself as I had been doing. The World Cup is very probably the single biggest sports event in the world, covered in London in 1966 by some 1,500 journalists. You can't cover it sitting still.

I made trips to Liverpool and Everton and to Wembley Stadium, where the London matches were played, and I walked a good part of the time. The first time I went to Wembley, I had my driver stop at the Green Man, a pub high on a hill overlooking the stadium, because I wanted to talk to the people in the pub before the game began. The driver parked the car and left it and I walked three blocks down the hill to the stadium just before the match started.

I was walking with a group of Liverpudlian soccer fans and I was discussing the upcoming match with them, after having had several pints of ale at the Green Man, and I had reached my seat in the press box before I suddenly realized that I had not thought of my heart at all, either on the long walk down the hill or in the climb up to my press-box seat.

I put my hand on my chest for a minute and my heart was pumping away steadily; I felt no distress, no angina. I decided then that I would have to go on as if I had never had a heart attack, within limits. I knew I wouldn't be making any block-long dashes to catch a bus, or trying to lift weights, but I felt sure that I could expect to do my job with no sweat. The heaviest thing a sports writer has to lift is a typewriter. I sold my old portable and bought a new Swiss-made machine that weighed only five or six pounds.

The night of the final match between England and West Germany, I worked virtually until dawn. I had got up early to go to Wembley for the match, watched what turned out to be an extraordinarily exciting game that went into two overtime periods, and forgotten my supposed unprejudiced stance to cheer lustily for England.

After the match (which England won 4–2), I made my way down under the stands to the dressing-room area and stood crowded in with hundreds of other reporters, watching TV interviews with the players, none of which was startling.

Leaving the stadium, I climbed back up that three-block hill to the Green Man, where a crowd lingered toasting the English victory, and I had a couple of beers there, looking for local color. I had been a little out of breath when I reached the top of the hill, but my heart didn't bother me and I didn't think about it at all. I was too engrossed in the story.

From there, I drove back into the heart of London to await the arrival of the victorious English team at their hotel, the Royal Garden, where a party was planned to go on most of the night. The crowd around the hotel was enormous, enthusiastic, and full of beer and I had to use force to push my way through to the lobby. No one was interested in my press credentials; the only pass that worked was physical force.

I spent two hours there, catching a rare word with some of the players as they came through the lobby on their way to the banquet hall, then I made my way back to my hotel. I had to walk, since my car and driver had disappeared by now, and it was a long walk at the end of a long day.

My mind was busy with the details of the story; I wouldn't have much time to write it, since the game had been played on a Saturday and the magazine goes to press Sunday night. I had to finish the story before I went to sleep and it would be a long and difficult story, because it was the first soccer competition I had ever covered.

I finally reached the hotel room and my wife was waiting for me, worried because I was late. I had forgotten my heart, but she hadn't.

"Are you all right?" she said when I came in. "I didn't know what had happened to you."

"All right?" I said. "Sure. Why shouldn't I be all right?"

"How is your heart?"

For the first time all day, I thought to myself how is your heart. As I sat down to the lightweight typewriter to do the story, I realized that my heart was fine, banging away steadily despite all the strain I had put on it.

"Fix me a scotch and soda," I said to Dorothy. "My heart is fine."

Then I wrote the story, which I finished about three in the morning and we went out to a club for more drinks and a steak dinner.

Chapter Four /

When I came back from England, I went directly into covering professional football, something I do for *Sports Illustrated* every fall. I was a little late getting started, so that I had to compress my travel schedule and work harder than usual for about six weeks, but I had no problems with my heart.

I had cut down on my visits to my doctor so that I saw him only once a month now, but I still took digitoxin and coumadin, although I was a bit apprehensive about the latter. On the road as much as I was, I was afraid that I might be involved in an auto accident or some other mishap which might inflict a severe cut. Unless someone knew that I was on coumadin, I could easily bleed to death.

I read the research material I could find on the drug and discovered that there is no clear-cut evidence that it prevents a recurrence of a heart attack. There are as many proponents of coumadin as there are those who say it has no appreciable effect, so I decided to quit the dosage entirely. I talked to Jerry about it and he agreed I could quit.

I haven't taken any since and I really don't think it is useful except immediately after a heart attack, in the first month or two. The side effects, other than bleeding, are not particularly pleasant anyway.

It was now some six months after I had had the heart attack, and, while I still found myself growing very tired in the late evening, I was no longer curtailing any of my normal activity. I drank socially, traveled, covered football games, and, to my sorrow, smoked.

For six months after the heart attack, I did not smoke. During that time, a close friend of mine in Los Angeles, who is about my age, had a heart attack and I wrote him a letter while he was in the hospital.

I told him about my recovery and about how well I felt and wound up the letter by saying that he had one big plus from the heart attack.

"At least, you'll have to stop smoking," I wrote smugly. "It's the hard way to stop, but it may be worth it in the long run."

All of which is very true, but I started smoking again. Not as much as I had. Before the attack, I was smoking two or three packs a day, sometimes more when I had to work eighteen or twenty hours closing a story.

I started smoking again while writing a story on a November football game in Dallas. I have forgotten which game it was now, but I remember that I had picked the Dallas Cowboys to win the National Football League championship that season. This was a key game and they got the hell kicked out of them.

I borrowed a cigarette from a friend in the press box, then another, then another, and by the time I got back to the hotel I had reached the point where I stopped at the cigarette stand and bought a pack.

I told myself that I would quit again in the morning, but I did not.

At this time I was taking as little exercise as possible. I walked slowly, took it easy climbing stairs, tried to rest as often as I could, and avoided sudden exertion of any kind. My electrocardiograms showed evidence of the damage done to my heart and Jerry did not think it advisable yet to try any exercise other than walking slowly.

I got through the football season well enough, with no ill effects when the Cowboys managed to blow their chance to win the NFL championship. Then I went to Houston on another fight story. While I was there, I decided that I would go through a famous heart clinic just to discover from another source what I could look forward to for the rest of my life.

I spent a day and a half taking tests, including the step test, in which the patient steps up and down on a small two-stair flight for a minute or so with the leads to an electrocardiograph attached to him, to determine the reaction of his heart to stress and, after, how quickly it recovers from the strain.

When I went into the office of the young doctor who had conducted most of the examinations, he had the data spread out on the desk in front of him. I looked curiously at the long EKG tapes, the x-rays, and the reports and wondered what was coming. His face was carefully non-commital.

"There is very clear evidence of your heart attack," he told me. "Your EKGs are abnormal and your heart recovers slowly from stress. It is enlarged quite a bit, which is usually what happens after a massive attack such as yours."

He held up a large x-ray to the light and traced the outline of my heart. I stared at it carefully, but I couldn't tell which was my heart. The only thing I was sure of was that I seemed to have a normal complement of ribs.

The doctor went on at some length, explaining the squiggles on the EKG and their significance and going over the other tests that had been made on me. Aside from my damaged heart, I seemed to be in pretty good shape, albeit a little heavier than I should have been. Sometimes, in the wake of a heart attack, the heart is unable to pump enough blood to allow other vital organs to function properly, but my heart, blown up as it was, seemed to be doing that well enough.

When he had finished and was returning all the documents to a large manila envelope, I said, "What are my prospects?"

"You can live a long time yet," he said, smiling. "People with scarred hearts are sometimes lucky for the heart attack. If they survive, it serves as a warning to take it easy and they live much longer than they might have with a later heart attack damaging an older heart."

"What do you mean by 'take it easy'?"

"I wouldn't advise you to have over one or two drinks

a day," he said. "No smoking at all, of course. Watch your diet and keep your weight down. I'll give you a low-cholesterol diet before you leave."

I wasn't exactly overjoyed at the number of drinks he proposed to limit me to. I could understand the restriction on cigarettes, although I hadn't been able to observe it, and the diet did not bother me, since I have never cared much for fatty foods or sweets anyway.

"How about exercise?" I asked then. "I've been going very slow, but I'd like to do something now."

He looked at me seriously for a long moment, then shook his head.

"I don't think so," he said. "Certainly not for the next year or so. And, even after that, I would suppose that the most you can expect is to be able to take leisurely walks. Nothing strenuous."

I walked out of the clinic into the hot, humid air of Houston and started to stroll slowly back to my hotel, which was about a half mile away. Coming out of the air-conditioned clinic, I felt the heat more than usual and I began to sweat quickly. There was no breeze and the sun beat down on my head with almost physical force, but I did not pay any attention to it.

I began to walk a little faster, very much aware of my heartbeat. For almost the first time since I had left the hospital, I was worried.

Of course I had not expected to get a clean bill of health. It had been almost exactly a year since the heart attack and I knew that I was certainly not fit to go a fast ten rounds with Muhammad Ali, but I had thought that I might be able to play golf, maybe even jog or swim a little.

But the doctor had been explicit about that when I had suggested it.

"Absolutely not," he said. "You have a damaged heart. It has about all it can do to keep going under normal living conditions. Any unusual strain could push it into fibrillation and failure."

Fibrillation is the rapid, fluttery beating of a heart that has lost its normal rhythm and it can be very quickly fatal if not corrected immediately.

By the time I got back to my hotel, I had rationalized my fear to some degree. After all, I had not been very active in participant sports for a long time, aside from an occasional round of golf and the rather haphazard exercise I had taken in the year or so just before my coronary.

So I took the elevator to the top of the Warwick Hotel, where the Warwick Club overlooks the Houston skyline, and had a couple of drinks to console myself. I decided that I would sacrifice my athletic career, but two drinks a day? There are some things doctors do not understand. I started to light a cigarette, then rubbed it out and threw away the pack.

I covered the fight that night in the Houston Astrodome. It was Muhammad Ali against Cleveland Williams and Ali won on a very quick knockout, so that I didn't have much of a story to write. I retired to a room in the Astrodome and began to write, and about halfway through the story I realized I was smoking. It is a conditioned reflex for most writers to smoke when they are doing a story; I had thrown away the pack at the Warwick Club, but by the time I realized I was smoking and writing, there were four or five butts in the ash tray on the table by my type-writer. I had bummed them without knowing it.

I would like to say that I put out that cigarette and never smoked another, but it would not be true. I quit once more after that, but it lasted only six months. I have tried to quit several other times. As someone once said, "It's easy to quit smoking. I have done so many times."

At any rate, I did not take any exercise for the next year. I performed all my regular duties as a writer for *Sports Illustrated* and finished three books that had been interrupted by the heart attack, but I spent an almost completely sedentary life. I didn't restrict myself to two drinks a day; I usually have several drinks at lunch and several before dinner and occasionally, on a story, I'll have more than that drinking with other writers, coaches, and athletes. I felt pretty good that year. I still got tired in the evening, but not the bone-weary exhaustion that had almost incapacitated me during the first year after the attack.

The drinking did not seem to have any effect, one way or the other. For some lucky reason, as I mentioned earlier, I have never had a hangover in my life; one doctor once told me it was because I have a very efficient liver. Another one told me it was because I have no guilt feelings about drinking. The first was a liver specialist and the second was a psychiatrist.

It was not an easy year, professionally. I had the usual six months of travel covering the professional football season and when that was over, I went to Geneva in the spring to cover a meeting of the International Olympic Committee, which was called to decide whether to allow South Africa to compete in the 1968 Olympic Games.

The committee decided, after long-drawn-out sessions, which were boring but not physically taxing to cover, to bar South Africa from the Olympic Games and I left Geneva on a long, grueling flight to Johannesburg, South Africa. Here I spent three weeks taking a long look at apartheid and its effect on sports in that country.

Joburg is, in many ways, a pleasant, civilized city. Its white inhabitants are friendly and convivial and anxious to help a visiting journalist. Unfortunately, the black population of South Africa lives under worse conditions than did the slave population of the South before the Civil War.

None of that has anything to do with my heart problem, other than that, during the three weeks I spent in South Africa, I was under continuing stress, something else the doctor in Houston had told me to avoid at all costs.

I could not accept the evidence the white South Africans were willing to let me see. I had to spend a good deal of time trying to get clandestine interviews with some of the dissident black population, which was neither easy nor designed to create a feeling of quiet repose in me.

To complicate matters more, I contracted a particularly virulent kind of dysentery, which prevented my sleeping a night through and interrupted my interviews with the upper-echelon South African whites no less than with the dissident Bantu. This malady continued all through my stay in South Africa. I lost some twenty pounds, which I needed to do, but I would not like to lose twenty pounds that way again.

I suppose that, if my heart had not been somewhat stronger than I thought at the time, I would not have survived an experience that had to do with the story only peripherally.

My photographer was an Englishman named Gerry Cranham, who is a wonderfully ingenious man at ferreting out good pictures and insinuating himself into a position where he can shoot them. While I was in Johannesburg, he spent almost two weeks with me, shooting everything he was allowed to shoot and quite a lot that the authorities would probably have preferred he not shoot.

In preparation for the story, the New York office suggested that Cranham take a picture of me in a setting that would be very clearly African. Gerry asked me if I had any ideas. I thought a picture of me racing for the men's room in the Johannesburg airport, under a sign saying "Johannesburg," would be appropriate, but he didn't take to that.

Some fifty or sixty miles out of Johannesburg is a national park in which the animals of the country are allowed to roam free. Gerry suggested that we take a trip out there. Actually, he first said that he thought a safari in Kenya would probably turn up the kind of picture we wanted, but I didn't think the home office would hold still for a charge of something like $10,000 for one picture of me.

So we hired a car and driver and went out to the park. It was a pleasant spot. As you entered, there was a large sign, with printing in Afrikaans and English, saying, "You are now entering lion country."

We bought tickets to enter lion country and were given a booklet to read before we drove through the gate. There were a few simple rules, designed to protect idiot tourists from killing themselves.

"Stay in your car, with the windows rolled up. Stay on the main roads. Under no circumstances get out of your car."

All of them seemed reasonable enough to me. We drove along, peering out the windows looking for lion, and soon enough we saw a pride resting under some trees off to the right about fifty yards. They were well off the main road.

"See if you can get closer to them," Gerry said to the driver, who looked at him askance.

"I can't leave the main road," he said. "Didn't you read the book?"

"There's a little road right there," Gerry said. "Turn on it."

The driver looked at me doubtfully, and I shrugged.

He looked back at Gerry, who was waving a few rand in his hand, and turned right. A rand is worth a little more than a dollar.

When we got within about ten yards of the lions, Gerry motioned to the driver to stop and we did. I must admit the lions were much more impressive up close than they had been from the main road. A big male with a dark mane lifted his head and looked at us through calm, yellow eyes, then put his head down again. It was early afternoon, hot and quiet, and most of the lions were asleep.

"I got the picture," Gerry said. He began adjusting several of his battery of cameras, focusing on the lions, and I watched with mild interest. I didn't think a picture of lions in their natural state would fit into a story on apartheid but that was Gerry's problem, not mine. I try not to have too much to do with the mental processes of photographers; it's an easy rule to follow.

I looked back at the lions, all of them now lying quietly, and marveled at how big a lion looks, up close. A big male is an enormously impressive animal, even asleep. The head is massive and the muscles in the forearms are huge. You can understand how a lion can break the back of an antelope with one swipe when you look at what he swipes with.

Gerry checked a couple of exposure meters and put a long lens on one of the cameras. He hadn't taken any pictures yet and I wondered what he was waiting for.

"All right," he said. "I think that's just about it. Get out and go over there and stand by them."

No one said anything for a little while. The driver was checking to make sure his window was rolled up as far as it would go and his door was locked. I was looking at the lions and trying to decide if I had heard Gerry correctly.

"Hurry," he said. Have you ever noticed that the English never say, "Hurry *up*"? What they say is just plain "Hurry." I thought about that then.

"Why?" I asked him, reasonably.

"For the picture," he said. "For the magazine. Do hurry before the buggers move off."

I thought about that for a few moments. I owe a great deal to the magazine, but I wasn't quite sure I owed that much.

"Are you afraid?" Gerry said, looking at me with surprise.

"Well," I said.

"They're *asleep*," Gerry said. "All you have to do is get out, walk over there by them, and I'll shoot the picture and we'll have just what they want. A picture of Tex Maule in Africa."

"You better shoot quick," the driver said nervously. "You might get him in a lion."

"Thank you," I said to the driver.

Gerry opened the door on the side away from the lions and pushed me. I tried to resist, but I thought maybe he's right and it will be a hell of a picture. I got out of the car, walked around, and took a step toward the lions and stopped.

Gerry had rolled down the window a few inches and had the long lens of one of the cameras aimed at the lions.

"Closer," he said. "Get closer."

For no reason that I can explain, I moved a few steps closer to the lions. I looked at them and they all seemed to be sleeping peacefully enough and I felt a little better. Up close, lions smell pretty bad.

I turned and smiled, hoping that Gerry would shoot in a hurry and not want to take another. That is a forlorn hope, of course. No photographer worth his salt ever shoots less than a hundred pictures if he needs one.

Gerry did not shoot. He rolled the window down a trifle more and said, "A little closer. I can't get you and the lions in focus."

The lions didn't seem to mind, so I moved another two steps closer. By now I was close enough to see the flies lighting on the whiskers of the big male. When a fly lit there, he twitched the whiskers and once he lifted his upper lip far enough for me to see his teeth. They were yellowish, as if he had smoked too much, and very big. Not especially sharp, but very big.

I turned back to Gerry again and he snapped a couple of quick shots and I started back to the car, but he motioned to me to stay where I was and, like an idiot, I did.

The lions were still quiet, but not for long.

As I turned to pose again, Gerry rolled his window down a little more and hollered, "Hah, hah, hah!" I froze, the big lion lifted his head, and I unfroze and sprinted back to the car and into it and rolled up my window.

"That was super," Gerry said. "Really super."

The big lion had stood up and he yawned and looked at the car.

Chapter Five /

In spite of this evidence that my heart was strong enough for at least mild exercise, I did not start to work out for several months. I stayed on in South Africa for two weeks, working on the story under the close and beady watch of a variety of agents of the South African government, then returned to London to write the story.

After I had been in London for a week, the South African version of *turista* disappeared. I had lost a good deal of weight and I was weak, but I was now beginning to consider exercise, since my heart seemed, to me, strong. I knew, from having discussed the matter with Jerry, that any kind of physical exercise using the big muscles of the chest and shoulders was not good for a heart patient and I knew from my reading on the subject that the two simplest and best exercises for the heart and lungs are swimming and jogging.

Both can be completely controlled in that the swimmer or jogger can go at whatever pace he chooses for as long as he chooses. Several of the editors on my magazine were joggers and it is much easier to find a place to run than a place to swim, so I began toying with the idea of doing some mild jogging when I returned to the States.

First, though, Dorothy and I had an appointment to go to Vevey, in Switzerland, for treatment by the late Dr. Paul Niehans. Dr. Niehans was an expensive and controversial doctor; we had heard about him from friends who had had his treatment and Dorothy was convinced that his particular regime would help strengthen my heart. I was doubtful, but willing to try it.

I suppose the most accurate description of the clinic Dr. Niehans operates in Vevey would be a rejuvenation center. The handsome hospital in which he treats the people who come to him in search of their youth is called Clinique La Prairie; if the Flower & Fifth Avenue is typical of hospitals, Dr. Niehans' place must rank at the very top for cleanliness, service, and meticulous care. Even after having taken the treatment, I'm not quite sure whether it is really effective or not. I am sure that it most certainly does not hurt.

When I arrived at the clinic, I was given the most thorough physical examination I had had up until that time. The examination, according to the attending physicians, was to determine just where I needed help. I had given them the history of my heart attack; Dr. W. Michel, the English-speaking chief doctor, assured me that Dr. Niehans' cellular therapy was perfectly safe for me to take.

The treatment is not legal in the United States, since it has not been proved effective to the satisfaction of the American Medical Association. In various forms, it is obtainable in most of Europe, including England.

Dr. Niehans has been using this method for relieving the symptoms of old age and for regenerating failing organs for some forty years and his clinical reports, made before scientific bodies in Europe, show some remarkable cures. Among his patients are Charles Chaplin, who became a father not long ago in his late seventies, and Spain's General Franco. A list of long-in-the-tooth entertainers and movie stars have visited the small clinic near Lake Geneva in the last twenty-odd years and while most of them do not boast publicly of having been there, they admit their debt to Dr. Niehans rather freely in private.

Niehans has almost retired by now; on the early June morning I checked in, he was in Madrid. No one said whether or not it was to treat Franco.

The treatment itself is simple enough. The exhaustive examinations indicate what cellular therapy you need and, on your first morning in the clinic, you get a series of shots designed to stimulate whichever of your organs need stimulation.

Niehans uses injections made up from cell soups from the appropriate organs of unborn lambs. The cells, supposedly, pep up the tired cells in the body and promote renewed vigor in the organs concerned. The effect is a delayed one; in a small booklet the clinic issues after you have spent your week of rest and seclusion there, Dr. Niehans writes that you do not begin to feel the benefit of his cellular therapy for at least three and a half months.

As a reminder, you also get a small white card which reads as follows:

TO MY PATIENTS!

Your organism has been given precious cells, which start to work after 3½ months. I beg you not to damage them in any way! Therefore:

NO x-rays without protecting the rest of the body.

NO shortwave treatment, no ultraviolet rays.

NO very hot hair drier.

NO bath cures in radioactive thermal stations.

NO sun baths, no Turkish baths, no sauna baths, no diathermy.

NO poisons, such as nicotine, concentrated alcohols.

NO drugs (if possible) and no hormones.

These instructions are for your whole life long.

Prof. Niehans
Burier / La Tour-de-Peilz
near Vevey (Switzerland)

My examination, unfortunately, revealed that I not only had a bad heart, but that there were some ten other areas in which my body was not operating at full speed. Dr. Michel told me the bad news on the night before I was to get the shots; I was considerably disturbed until I learned by checking with other patients that eleven malfunctioning organs was about par for the course. In my case, this included the liver, kidneys, and gall bladder, among others.

At ten the next morning, Dr. Michel, accompanied by

a nurse and a rolling table loaded with cell cultures and hypodermic needles all about the size of a knitting needle, walked in cheerfully and asked me to roll over on my stomach.

When I had, the nurse bared my bottom and Dr. Michel zapped me eleven times, changing needles between each shot. After the last shot, he patted me on the shoulder and advised me to lie on my stomach for the next thirty minutes, advice which I really did not need.

For the next two days, I had to stay in bed constantly, getting up only very briefly to go to the john. The hospital diet was mild but good enough; when I had first seen the examining physician, he had told me that for me, with a heart condition, smoking was poison. Since cigarettes were banned in the hospital in any case, that was no problem.

Surprisingly, after two days, I was allowed a half bottle of wine with my evening meal, at an extra charge, of course. After the opening shots, the only treatment was rest; I stayed in the hospital for seven days and six nights and was not allowed to take a walk until the fifth day. This, it was explained to me, was to give the delicate unborn lamb cells a chance to survive and do their work.

If the treatment did nothing else for me, it helped me quit smoking again. When I drove away from Vevey, some $3,000 poorer but rested, I was off cigarettes and I felt much better than I had in quite a while.

My wife and I drove across France to the Channel on our way back to London and by the time we stopped in Rouen for the night, I had developed an itchy rash all over my backside. I figured that I must be allergic to lamb and tried to ignore it but it was worse in the morning and I called the clinic.

"That is a normal reaction," Dr. Michel told me soothingly. "If it doesn't go away in a week, please call again."

It went away in about three days. I've never had any allergic reaction to lamb taken by mouth.

One of the temporary restrictions placed on me when I left the clinic was on exercise.

"You may walk," Dr. Michel said. "But no strenuous exercise of any kind. These new cells are very delicate. I would suggest you wait at least three months before you do anything more than stroll."

The electrocardiogram which had been taken at the clinic showed the damage of my heart attack, but the doctors there felt that, after the three-month waiting period, mild exercise would not be harmful to me. Indeed, they thought that it might be advisable, especially since my heart, presumably strengthened by whatever unborn-lamb heart cells had augmented it, should be better able to accommodate a heavier load.

I had taken the shots on June 3, 1968; on September 1, two and a half years after my heart attack, I began a careful program which included a little jogging.

In the meantime, we had returned to the United States and, after a brief stay in New York, I had set out on my annual trip to the training camps of the teams in the National Football League.

I very carefully avoided x-rays, shortwaves, ultraviolet rays, bath cures in radioactive thermal stations, sun baths, Turkish baths, sauna baths, diathermy, drugs, and hormones. Hair driers were no problem, but poisons were not so easy, especially concentrated alcohols.

Since, for one reason or another, I spend quite a bit of time in bars talking to disreputable people like sports writers, publicity men, club owners, and retired football players, I found it very difficult to avoid concentrated alcohol. For two months, I drank plain soda.

Plain soda is fine, mixed with scotch, which dampens its tendency toward excessive effervescence. Taken without a mixer, it tends to inflate the drinker until he burbles constantly, like a sleeping volcano. After two months on plain soda, I figured the unborn lamb cells had grown up enough for a beer or two. Beer is not concentrated alcohol, anyway.

So I changed from soda to beer, but beer is a tough tipple to stick with through a long night, especially after a protracted afternoon. I gained about twenty pounds coddling the lamb cells before I decided that they were old enough for an occasional vodka and tonic or scotch and water. I was still anti-soda then.

At first, each time I sipped a scotch or a vodka, I could feel the cells curdling. I felt very good, even with the paunch I had acquired drinking the beer, but my physical euphoria was diminished by the guilt I felt for what I was doing to my lamb cells. For the first two or three drinks, I worried about the cells, then I thought the hell with it, they're probably old enough by now to drink.

By the time I got back from covering all the clubs in the NFL, I was host to several million alcoholic lamb cells, but I still felt good and I wasn't smoking.

My wife had been observing me thoughtfully, checking to see if my hair was turning darker or growing thicker or if I walked with a springier step or a few other things and she seemed a trifle disappointed when I came back from California, my last stop on the scouting tour.

"It's just about three and a half months now," I told her. "God help you next week."

"Have you been drinking?"

"Not much," I said. "Not enough to hurt."

It was late August and I really had a couple of weeks to go before all the little lamb cells turned to and began to work. In the meantime, I had to write the scouting reports on the pro clubs for the special pro football issue of the magazine. This is a difficult, plodding job and one afternoon, trying for the umpteenth time to find a new way to say that team X would have a hard time trying to limit my maiden aunt Maisie to twenty pass completions with a secondary defense composed of four drunken lamb cells, I got up from my typewriter and walked through the halls.

I stopped to talk to my friends in every office on the twentieth floor of the Time & Life Building, a procedure most writers follow in trying to avoid writing. One of them was smoking and I looked at his cigarette longingly.

I don't really know about the other people who smoke, but I have found, during the two rather short periods I have managed to quit smoking, that it is totally untrue that, once you have quit for two weeks, you have it made.

I never have it made. Every morning, after I have had breakfast, I want a cigarette. Every night, after dinner, I want a cigarette. At lunch, I drink vodka and tonic and seldom eat and I want a cigarette. When I write—especially when I write—I want a cigarette.

I didn't start smoking until I was thirty. I was on a merchant ship, bound for the coast of Japan, with provisions to support our invasion. The war ended when we were two weeks beyond the Panama Canal and all of us on the S.S. *Sturdy Beggar* thought we would turn around and come home. What we were carrying was oil used by destroyers to set up smoke screens for the landings; with no landings in prospect, it seemed reasonable that we would come home.

But we went on to Japan and on the way, we stopped in Manila Bay for sixty-four days. The oil was carried in drums and we had several thousand drums and the old man—the captain—had said we would not be going home until we had discharged all of the oil. We discharged ten drums in sixty-four days; there was a very limited market for fog oil in Manila at the time.

From there we went on to Yokosuka, in Japan. We sold the fog oil to the Japanese for diesel fuel and after we had been discharging for a few days the harbor was secured from air attack. All the tugs were emitting smoke screens, and so was I.

Cigarettes were six cents a pack on the ship and a dollar a pack on the black market in Japan just after the war. I could buy two cartons of cigarettes for a buck twenty, get on the train for Tokyo in Yokosuka and sell them for twenty bucks by the time I reached Tokyo. It made for very cheap weekends.

But it was still boring sitting for another two months in Japan while we discharged drums into bumboats at a painfully slow rate. One day I tried a cigarette on the theory that if the Japanese, who didn't have any money, would spend a dollar a pack for smokes, they must have something I didn't know about.

The first cigarette made me dizzy and I didn't really begin to like them until we were on the way home—two months at sea with nothing at all to do.

By the time we docked in New Orleans, about five months after the war had ended, I was hooked.

So, searching for the right way to say what eventually turned out to be the wrong thing, I borrowed a cigarette, thinking that I would just smoke the one to demonstrate to myself how little I really needed a cigarette. I was right. I smoked just one that day, but the way was open again and the lamb cells, if any of them had survived the vodka and scotch, were as long lost as Little Bo Peep's charges.

I fought the good fight until the season started and I was doing a story under a deadline. I knew that I had lost when I bought a pack of cigarettes. As long as you're still borrowing, you can delude yourself into thinking that you're not really smoking again. Once you walk up to the counter and buy a pack, you're dead. Dead. A peculiarly appropriate word to use.

Well, at this point I was full of dying lamb cells and I was drinking and smoking and, because of my experiment with drinking beer and all I had eaten while I was off cigarettes, forty-five pounds overweight.

I was in San Francisco, on a story about why the San Francisco Forty-Niners always look wonderful and play something less than that. I was at their training camp, talking to Lou Spadia, who is the general manager of the club. Lou runs every day, up to three miles.

I was very much interested in running. Andrew

Crichton, a rather emaciated looking man who serves brilliantly as a copy editor—senior editor, in his case—for *Sports Illustrated*, has been running a long time. He has had almost every nonfatal ailment known to mankind. Yet he is an obnoxiously cheerful, charming human being.

He runs any where from five to innumerable miles a day and he runs in the Boston Marathon every year, finishing back in the ruck behind the women who are striking a blow for liberation and the fourteen-year-old boys who are simply being a pain in the ass. But he finishes. And he is lean. I remember when he was not lean.

He had been after me to run for some time, a proposition I entertained enthusiastically as long as it was in the indeterminate future. Now I saw Spadia running and I decided that I had to make a decision. Run or else. I did not try to imagine what the *or else* would be. And I had read a book on running by Dr. Kenneth Cooper, who was the physical fitness director for the United States Air Force.

Chapter Six /

Dr. Cooper's book is called *Aerobics;* for the next three years it might have just as well been called the Bible, for me. I worked out my running schedule by it, improved with it, and, in effect, lived by it in both senses of the word.

I had already read the book by the time I reached the Forty-Niner training camp, so I knew that Dr. Cooper's test for fitness is to discover how far you can go—running, walking, crawling, or any combination of the three —in twelve minutes. I decided that I would take the test while Spadia was doing his daily three miles on the track at the University of California at Santa Barbara, where the Forty-Niners do their preseason training.

I borrowed gear from the Forty-Niner equipment

manager—sweat suit, jockstrap, and cleated low-cuts. Before we went out on the track, I weighed myself—215 flabby pounds. I had weighed about 205 at the time of the attack.

As we walked to the track, Lou told me about his own conversion to running. He had started with the Forty-Niners when the club was organized by Tony and Vic Morabito, two San Francisco trucking magnates. Both of them had died of heart attacks in the previous five years.

"I hadn't thought much about my heart until Vic died," Lou said. "But when you lose two close friends in a few years, you begin to wonder about yourself, so I had a thorough checkup. My heart was okay, but I was overweight, I didn't exercise and I smoked too much. The doctor suggested that I quit smoking, start walking, and lose weight."

That had been two years before. Spadia, on the morning we ran together, was trim and fit-looking. He appeared years younger than his forty-odd and when we reached the track and he began to run, I found out quickly enough that he was a century younger than I.

"I'll go the first half mile with you, then slow down," I said, confidently. "I don't want to work too hard at first. I figure it'll take me a couple of months or so to work up to two miles."

The track at Santa Barbara is the conventional quarter-mile oval; we started running in the middle of the home straight and by the time we had reached the end of the first turn, I was finished. I had run something less than two hundred yards and I was gasping desperately for breath. When your heart and lungs are as far out of condition as mine were then, you feel as if it is impossible to draw a deep enough breath.

I sucked in air as deeply as I could, but I hit a barrier in my chest so that I could not inhale nearly enough. I stopped running and walked around the track, then started at a gentle jog again.

I quit that day after an inglorious half mile, most of which I negotiated at a slow, wind-broken walk. Lou ran some two miles during the time I walked, rested, trotted a few steps, and rested again.

As we walked back to the gym to shower and change, I asked Lou how long it had taken him to learn to run so easily.

"A year," he said. "At least a year. You got to take it easy. But if you stick to it, it's worth it. I had my annual checkup last week. I always ask doc to check my heart especially, so he takes not only the regular electrocardiogram with the gear on my arm, but he tests the blood pressure in my legs, too. He said I had the best circulation and blood pressure in my legs he had seen in a long time, even in patients younger by ten years."

As we dressed, I told him about Crichton and his yearly run in the Boston Marathon.

"I'd settle for being able to run two miles without stopping," I said. "But I doubt that I can make even that, Lou. Not after today."

"What does your doctor say?" Lou asked.

"Take it easy," I replied.

"So walk, don't run," Lou suggested.

The next morning, my legs were sore as boils, but I went out to the track again. This time I decided I would see just how fit I was by taking Dr. Cooper's test—going as far as I could go in twelve minutes.

The test is based on the amount of oxygen your body can use during all-out effort; the fitter you are, the more oxygen you can utilize, the farther and faster you can go. Dr. Cooper has reduced the complicated testing techniques of the laboratory to a simple physical test.

At my age then—fifty-three—any distance under eight-tenths of a mile meant that I was in very poor condition. To qualify as in excellent condition, I would have to run a mile and a half or more.

When we reached the track, Lou went off at his steady, easy pace while I waited and watched the sweep hand of my wrist watch. I started my test as it passed zero, running much slower than I had the day before, determined to at least exceed eight-tenths of a mile. The next category above very poor is poor and I was willing to settle for that.

The going was no easier than it had been the day before and it was made more painful because my legs ached after a few steps. I ran about fifty steps, then slowed to a walk, already puffing. I decided I would try to do the whole thing at the Boy-Scout pace—fifty steps trotting, fifty walking.

Lou passed me early on, finishing his first lap, then a runner in a disreputable-looking red sweat suit went by Lou at what to me seemed to be sprinter's speed. I barely noticed him; by now, only about four minutes into the testing time, I was laboring heavily and I began to run twenty-five steps and walk seventy-five. Three minutes later, I settled for a brisk walk. When the twelve minutes had passed, I had managed to cover only a few yards more than a half mile.

Even by Dr. Cooper's generous standards, that qualified me, as near as I could estimate, as moribund. I walked slowly for a few minutes, mindful of Dr. Cooper's warning that you must cool down after exercise as well as warm up before it.

I sat on the edge of the track and watched Lou jogging around and suddenly realized I knew the sprinter in ragged red who was lapping him regularly. It was Crichton.

Andy stopped after another fast lap and pulled off his sweats. He stopped by me and I asked him what he was doing in Santa Barbara.

"Vacation," he said, and his breathing was much easier than mine, although he must have run a couple of miles by then. "You decided to start running?"

"No," I said. "I just decided to stop running."

"I'm gonna do five now," Andy said. "Wait till I get through."

"What were you doing before?"

"Warming up."

He set off again, going even faster now. Unlike most distance runners, Andy runs on his toes. He looks light as a feather, going with a long, easy stride which seems effortless. I watched him sourly while Lou finished and sat down by me.

"Who's that?" he asked.

"Crichton," I said. "The guy I was telling you about."

Spadia watched Andy breeze by and shook his head.

"Must be nice to be young," he said. "Wish I had started at his age."

"You haven't had a good look at him," I said. "He's older than you are." I'm not sure that is true, but Andy is in his forties, anyway.

"How far is he going?" Lou asked.

"Five," I said. "He was just warming up for two."

"Oh," Lou said and we watched Crichton in silence until he had finished his five miles, which did not take long.

Andy finished by sprinting the last quarter mile, then jogged another half and came over to us.

"Really feels good running here," he said, still not out of breath. "Funny how much difference clean air makes. You can't breathe half the time in New York."

I introduced him to Spadia and we walked back to the gym together. My legs had started to stiffen and Lou and Andy had to slow down to match their pace to my hobble.

Crichton is an exuberant, enthusiastic man, an incurable optimist for himself—and for others. He asked me again if I had started a running program and I shook my head.

"I was thinking about it," I said. "But I guess I'm too old. Hell, I didn't even like running when I was in school. God knows how long it would take me to get to where I could run a quarter of a mile, let alone two. I guess I'll stick to walking."

"It's not that bad," Andy said cheerfully. "I couldn't run any better than you can when I started."

"How long ago was that?" Lou asked him. "When you were eighteen?"

"No," Andy said, and laughed. "About seven years ago. I weighed about 175 and I hadn't taken any exercise in years. I was doing track for the magazine and I covered a marathon and I thought to myself, that looks like fun. So I started running and, two years later, I ran in a marathon myself and finished. It took a long time, but I finished."

Lou looked at him sourly. Runners, from the slowest jogger on the block to international class marathoners, look with undisguised envy at anyone faster.

"All I want is exercise," he said.

"That's all I wanted to begin with," Andy said. "But it grows on you."

"Not me," I said. I could feel blisters on my feet now.

"Hey," Andy said. "Don't quit so soon. You'll be surprised how fast you come around."

"Maybe you," I said. "Not me. Not with my heart."

"I don't know about that," Andy said. "I guess you better check with your doctor."

Which, of course, is excellent advice. *No* one, repeat *no* one, should begin an exercise program without medical clearance. A young man might get away with it, but once you have passed thirty, then medical clearance is an absolute must. And at fifty-plus, two years after a massive heart attack, I should have had an exhaustive physical before exercising.

Of course, I had had that kind of examination in Houston and had been told that I should take only very light exercise. I thought about that now and considered mentioning it as an excuse for giving up jogging before I started, but for some reason, I didn't. I suppose no one particularly likes admitting a weakness; certainly I don't.

"I'll try for a while," I said all at once. I'm still not quite sure why I committed myself. I think I wanted to prove the doctors wrong and I know I was tired of taking care of myself as if I were a semi-invalid.

We had reached the gym by now and Andy left to go back to the house he had rented in Santa Barbara. I stood under a hot shower for a long time, trying to ease the ache in my legs. I had blisters on both feet and I was desperately tired and I could not imagine ever being able to run as far as a mile.

I looked down at the volleyball-sized pot belly I had accumulated in the last couple of years and looked at Lou; his stomach was flat as a board and he looked strong and healthy. I thought of Andy, going easily and smoothly for five miles and finishing without taking a deep breath. I remembered the agony I had had trying to breathe after only a couple of hundred yards.

I asked Lou if he had had trouble breathing at first.

"Sure," he said. "I wasn't any better than you. I guess no one is."

"Did your legs kill you?"

"They still do, sometimes," he said. "But I feel a hundred times better than I did before I started running. And I never run out of gas in the evening. Hell, my wife says my disposition has improved, too."

"All from running?"

"I'm not doing anything else different."

That evening Dorothy and I had dinner with Andy and Elizabeth, his wife. We talked about running for the whole evening, somewhat to the disgust of our wives. I found the conversation fascinating; it was the first time I had heard the gospel of jogging, but it was not to be the last. Indeed, in time I became as much of a bore on the subject as Dorothy considered Andy to be that night.

By the time the evening ended, I had made a firm decision to begin training immediately. One thing Andy said I found unbelievable, but months later I discovered it to be true.

In telling me, at considerable length, about the joys of running, he said, "One day you'll be running along and suddenly you'll discover that you're not even thinking about breathing. Your legs may ache a little, but the breathing won't be any problem. If you run far enough and long enough, eventually you reach the point where it will be almost impossible to run yourself out of breath."

I started to argue with him, then I remembered the way he had run that afternoon and I shut up. Even Lou, going at his rather stately pace, had run three miles and finished without breathing hard. I could not conceive of myself doing that, but I was in no position to dispute anyone with Andy's very evident expertise.

We spent a good deal of the time talking about proper equipment and I think this is one of the few enjoyable aspects of beginning a running program.

The next day, Dorothy and I returned to Los Angeles. It was mid-August and very hot and we stayed in one of the cottages at the Beverly Hills Hotel. I went off as soon as we had registered and visited a sporting goods store, where I bought running shorts, a sweat suit, and a pair of running shoes. The shoes turned out to be much too heavy, but at the time I felt that they gave me a rather professional look.

Late in the afternoon, I put on all my gear and walked across Sunset Boulevard for a run in the small park across from the hotel. The equipment didn't make much difference. My legs were still sore and my breath short and, if anything, I went slower than I had the day before. But I felt better in running gear.

Old ladies walking their dogs and old gentlemen sitting on park benches eyed me doubtfully as I slogged along at a fast walk or a minimal jog trot, but I paid them no attention. I was too concerned with catching my breath and, going by myself now, I was strongly aware of my heart. I had read of the pain exercise can cause a damaged heart and I monitored my heart second by second, ready to stop at the first twinge.

I had no twinges, even though my breathing was short and labored. I have never had a twinge running, although my chest has felt tight and constricted often enough.

I was extraordinarily fortunate, when I look back. I violated the one really cardinal rule of exercise for post-cardiac patients by beginning without my doctor's clearance. I survived but I can't say too strongly that no one should begin the way I did.

Upon my return from Switzerland after visiting the Niehans Clinic, I had gone to Jerry for a checkup and told him that I was considering light exercise. He agreed that it might be beneficial, if I took it very easy. During the next two and half years, I saw Jerry regularly for checkups and had two annual checkups at Time-Life, Inc. and I told Jerry and the Time-Life doctors that I was jogging. They approved, since I showed no ill effects.

Chapter Seven /

If there is a more difficult place in the world for joggers than New York City, I would be hard put to name it. You can run outdoors on the streets if you don't mind getting up at about six in the morning to avoid the fumes of the traffic and the jeers of the populace. You can run in Central Park, but the air pollution there is no better than on the roads and the people no kinder. Or you can run indoors, at one of the YMCAs or at the New York Athletic Club.

I picked the West Side YMCA for a number of reasons, the principal one being that Crichton and several other *Sports Illustrated* staffers work out there.

I wasn't anxious to demonstrate my turtle pace and deplorable condition to friends, but it is much easier to run in company than it is to run alone. As long as we ran indoors, I *was* running in company.

The indoor track at the West Side Y is a balcony over the basketball court. Most indoor YMCA tracks are built the same way, although this is one of the better ones with a good composition surface and banked turns, so that your feet and legs are not punished as severely as they would be on the hardwood tracks you find in some Ys.

Then, of course, it is a good deal cheaper to join a Y than to buy membership in an athletic club. In New York, a senior membership costs $150 a year; transportation, towel charges, and tips add another $150, more or less, so that my first year's jogging cost about $300, plus the cost of equipment.

I suppose I went through the same thing most beginners do as far as equipment is concerned. I started with a very simple cotton T-shirt and white cotton shorts, with the heavy, thick-soled shoes I had bought in Los Angeles. I now wear nylon running gear, because it washes and dries much more quickly than the cotton.

I kept the heavy shoes for a couple of months, which was a mistake.

I started what I suppose you might call my formal training program on September 1, 1968. I had worked out sporadically for the previous two weeks, in California and at home, jogging in place, but on the first of September, I began keeping a log of how many miles I had gone and how long it had taken me.

At first I listed the date, the number of miles, the time, aerobic points earned, and my weight before and after running. Aerobic points are a measure of the amount of exercise you have taken devised by Dr. Cooper, who has published a table of aerobic values for all kinds of exercise.

In order to reach and retain a reasonable degree of physical fitness, Dr. Cooper recommends that you should earn at least thirty points a week. I had decided to jog five times a week, since he recommends no less than three days work a week, with four better and five better still. Since I knew I couldn't put in any long distances, or go fast enough to earn points quickly, I set my goal at two miles in under twenty-four minutes, enough to make six points a day.

My notes for the first day show that I went two miles in twenty-four minutes and twenty seconds, which earned me only four points. If I had been able to cut that time by twenty-one seconds, I would have made the six, but by the time I was on the last lap of the two miles (or the forty-eighth lap of the tiny Y track), all I was interested in doing was finishing alive. I settled for the four points very happily.

I discovered another of the advantages of training at the Y when I stepped onto the track at a little after one in the afternoon that first day. In my running outfit, I looked rather like a large pear supported by two matchsticks; most of the 215 pounds I was carrying seemed to be between my waist and my hips, so that when I stripped and looked down at my belly, my bellybutton peered back up at me.

I was naturally a bit reluctant to go on the track after I had dressed, since I had a mental image of dozens of fleet, sinewy athletes staring contemptuously at me as they went by.

But the fleet, sinewy athletes do not, thank the lord,

train on indoor tracks which go twenty-four laps to the mile. They can't run fast enough on such a tiny oval. So when I stepped gingerly onto the track and began walking a few laps to warm up, I discovered happily enough that I wasn't the fattest one there by quite a few pounds.

There were several middle-aged men carrying paunches at least as large as mine, paddling around the track sedately. For a few minutes, before I began running myself, I even entertained the dream that I would not be the slowest man on the track, either.

I was, though. It is surprising how slow another jogger looks when you are on the outside edge of the track, walking along trying to look athletic. Once you have begun to jog yourself, in the beginning, it is just as surprising how fast he seems to be going when you try to keep up with him.

I had no idea that first day how I would do the two miles. I knew that I could not run the entire distance; I had found out to my sorrow how impossible that was for me when I had run in Santa Barbara.

I thought that if I went slowly enough, I might manage to do a half mile before I had to walk. Actually, I did six laps, or a quarter of a mile, then slowed to a walk, panting painfully.

There are traffic rules on an indoor track which are much more rigidly observed than the rules of the road, as I discovered at once. I had just started walking when a pot-bellied little man with white hair trundled around me and shouted, "Track!" in my ear at the top of his voice. I smiled and waved at him, a bit surprised that he should say something so obvious, but as I did someone behind me yelled, "Track!" again and shot by.

Finally Crichton, who had been zipping around the outside of the track at a fearsome pace, slowed up and explained to me that they were not greeting me as a new recruit.

"You run on the inside and walk on the outside," he said. "When they holler track, it's just a polite way to say 'Get the hell out of the way.'"

These indoor tracks are only eight to ten feet wide, so rigid traffic control is a necessity. I skipped to the outside of the track and walked six laps before I began to jog again and moved in on the pole.

My jogging pace was not a great deal faster than my walk, but as long as you give the appearance of trotting instead of walking, you are free to stay in the inside lane.

After the first day, I decided that I would have to figure out a graduated system of walking and jogging, designed to cut back on walking time and add to running time gradually. The two weeks haphazard running had not helped me at all; I felt as tired and discouraged after that first afternoon at the Y as I had in Santa Barbara.

The next day I decided I would jog four laps and walk eight, alternately, for the first week and the going was easier. I finished my two miles in twenty-five minutes and forty-nine seconds, but I was able to walk down the two flights of stairs to the locker room without stopping to rest twice, as I had the day before. And I still made my four points.

I had been afraid that I would be shunned by the competent runners at the Y, but I found out immediately that no one cares how fast you go. Joggers, from the best to the worst (me), are friendly and helpful. Crichton went out of his way to be helpful and total strangers, passing me time after time on the small track, offered words of encouragement.

By the end of the first week I had managed to do two miles in twenty-three minutes and fifty-five seconds once, but I discovered, to my dismay, that despite my exercise I had gained two pounds. My belly still bounced in counter-rhythm to my stride when I jogged and my bellybutton still looked up at me accusingly when I looked down.

Like most people, I had thought that the exercise, especially in the heat of early September, would melt pounds off, but that is a fallacy. Actually, going two miles at my snail's pace, I was very probably burning up only a little more than a hundred calories per session; the exercise and the knowledge that I was taking it encouraged me to add more than that to my regular diet.

I would lose a pound a workout, but that was, of course, only water loss, which I put back on as soon as I reached the nearest bar and gulped down a beer. The cold beer tasted marvelous, but one or two beers more than made up for the hundred-odd calories I had used as fuel for the jog.

At the end of the week, I went to Cleveland to cover a Cleveland Browns football game and ran at the Cleveland Y. The track there is twenty-two laps to the mile; I ran on it in the early morning, after having done my sparkling sub-twenty-four-minute two miles the day before and finished in something over twenty-six minutes, totally exhausted. I decided that they must have mismeasured the track, but I have found since that my times away from New York are consistently slower than they are at home. I'm not quite sure why this is—probably a combination of fatigue and tension brought on by travel and the fact that I cannot pace myself as well on a strange track.

It is barely possible that the time I spend drinking with other sports writers on the road contributes something to it.

After a week, I was still jogging four laps and walking eight in each half mile, but when I returned to New York, I changed the ratio to five and seven, with no ill effect.

During the next three weeks, I added a lap of jogging and deducted a walking lap each week until, at the beginning of October, a month after starting the workouts, I was running eight laps and walking only four. On October 1, I finished the two miles in about twenty-three and a half minutes and felt reasonably well doing it. My breathing was still difficult, but not nearly as labored as it had been; my heart thumped noisily for a while after I finished running, but I had no chest pain.

Where I had pain was in my knees. This began after I had been working out for about ten days. At first, my knees were sore but not acutely painful and I supposed that this was just part of the general soreness of my legs. But as the days went by and the muscular soreness subsided, my knees got worse and worse.

I was determined not to miss a day of jogging, so I ran through the pain every day I went to the Y. On the very bad days, I had trouble getting out of bed in the morning and before I went to the track I would take a couple of aspirin tablets to deaden the pain a little.

The pain would be intense as I began to jog, then die down after about a half mile. As long as I jogged, it would be bearable, but it would return when I walked.

The bad knees helped, in one way. Since it hurt more to walk than to run, I decided to run a full mile before walking and found, to my surprise, that I could. Now I would run a mile, slowly, then do the second mile walking four laps and jogging eight in each half. I was still wearing the very heavy, thick-soled shoes I had bought in Los Angeles.

The pain was most severe just at the top of the knee-cap, but my knees hurt on both sides of the joint, as well. Early in October, the pain was so severe and the joints so stiff that one day I could not force my foot into the running shoe. My shoes fit snugly and required an effort to put on, but it hurt so much for me to push my foot into the shoe that I had to give up.

I knew that if I could get on the track and jog awhile, the pain would ease and my stiffness would loosen up, but there is a rule against running barefoot at the West Side Y.

I finally solved the problem by buying a pair of judo slippers for a couple of dollars. These are very light canvas slippers which have almost no padding in the sole, so that they are useless for road running, but they worked very well on the smooth surface of the indoor track.

The first time I ran in the judo slippers, I did the two miles almost a minute faster than I had run it before. My knees hurt, but the pain seemed to subside much more quickly than it had before I changed shoes, so from then on I ran in the judo shoes. For a while, the bottom of my feet were sore from the lack of padding, but that was not nearly as uncomfortable as aching knees.

The improvement was only temporary, unfortunately. Running in judo slippers, I found that I could go faster, but the pain in my knees persisted for a long time. I finally checked with one of the team doctors in the National Football League to find out if there was anything seriously wrong with me.

"How long has it been since you did any real running?" he asked me.

"Lord knows," I said. "Maybe thirty years."

"So your ligaments were as stiff as dried leather," he said. "They're stretching now and the stretching hurts. When they loosen up enough, the pain will probably go away."

"How long will that take?"

He shrugged. "You can't tell," he said. "It depends on your age, your tissues, and how much you run."

"I don't know about my tissues," I said. "I'll probably keep on running two miles a day. And I'm not young. So what do you think? Another week or another month?"

"It could be another year," he said cheerfully.

"Thanks," I told him.

Actually, the knees hurt off and on for about three months. By October 24, a little less than two months after I had begun jogging, I was able, for the first time, to run two miles without stopping. On that day, my knees were very bad and I went two because I did not want to let them stiffen up by walking. I went slowly and did the two miles in a little less than twenty-one minutes; three days earlier, I had just broken twenty minutes and just gone under 190 pounds.

So I was some twenty-two pounds lighter and five minutes faster than I had been. I felt better already, except for the knees, and I had begun to develop the habit of jogging. I think the diary of running I kept contributed a great deal to the continuity of the effort; by the end of October, I had reached the point where I would go to almost any lengths to avoid missing a scheduled workout.

My heart had not bothered me at all. When I had started running my pulse rate was around ninety beats a minute; now it had been reduced to the low eighties, still not good, but better than I had expected so soon.

Chapter Eight /

By November, I had established an almost invariable routine. I jogged Tuesday through Saturday and rested Sunday and Monday, a schedule dictated more by my workweek and drink habits than by anything else.

The editorial workweek at *Sports Illustrated* begins on Thursday and goes through Monday; the longest day is Sunday, when the magazine goes to press. I was in the middle of the professional football season, which meant that usually I would leave New York on Thursday to go to a game somewhere in the country, and return to New York either late Sunday night or early Monday morning. Sunday, with a game to cover, I found it very difficult to find time for running. On Monday, after a long night of drinking and writing or traveling, I felt the need of rest.

Occasionally on the road, I would be unable to get to a YMCA to run; I ran in place in my hotel room then, figuring 800 steps with my left foot the equivalent of a mile. I arrived at that figure by counting steps while running at the West Side Y. The number of steps varied from day to day with my running speed; the faster I ran, the fewer steps to the mile since my stride stretched out a bit.

Another of the advantages of a YMCA membership for a jogger is that your membership card gives you visiting privileges at any YMCA in the country. By the end of my first year of jogging, for instance, I had run in YMCAs in Cleveland, Minneapolis, Houston, Green Bay, Milwaukee, Baltimore, San Francisco, Los Angeles, Miami, Westchester (California), Long Beach, Thousand Oaks, San Diego, Santa Barbara, and St. Louis.

I had also run at the Duke of York Headquarters in the Kings Road in London and in the Astrodome in Houston. I had jogged across Hampstead Heath and through the streets of Chelsea in London, as well as along the banks of the Thames.

My weight had gone from 215 to 166½ and my waist from forty to thirty-three, a change which wiped out an entire wardrobe. My wife and daughter thought I was too thin and looked older and some of my friends, if they had not seen me for some time, inquired anxiously about my health, but I felt better than I had in years.

Just before the end of my first year of jogging, I tried the twelve-minute fitness test again; originally, in Santa Barbara, I had barely passed the half-mile mark, running outdoors on a quarter-mile track, where you should be able to beat your indoor times.

I had avoided testing myself for twelve minutes, although I knew that I had moved steadily toward good conditioning. In running two-mile stints during most of 1969, I checked on my time as I went through a mile and a half and it had gradually come closer and closer to twelve minutes. Within six months I had passed through fair on Dr. Cooper's scale, running a mile and a quarter in twelve minutes while running a total of two miles. I didn't try an all-out twelve-minute test until I was reasonably sure I could qualify as being in good condition.

This time, running indoors at the West Side Y on the twenty-four-laps-to-a-mile track, I ran a hundred yards farther than a mile and a half in twelve minutes and felt better finishing than I had a year earlier after a half mile.

My time for two miles, figuring from the first time that I was able to run two miles without stopping, dropped from 24 minutes and 28 seconds to 15 minutes 53.4 seconds; my three-mile time went from 26:29.0 to 24:51.4. The improvement at three miles was not as dramatic as for the shorter distances because I did not start running three miles at a clip until I was in pretty good condition. I ran three miles for the first time in early February, after five months training.

By the end of the first year, I had run a total of 714 miles and spent 105 hours, 17 minutes, 4.2 seconds on the track, plus probably three times as much time boring people talking about it.

After three months, I bought a stopwatch and a lap counter; both are useful in trying to avoid the boredom which accompanies indoor running. Running as slowly as I did, I certainly could not compete with any other runner on the track and the stopwatch allowed me to compete with myself. The tallier, a small gadget which keeps count as you push a button after each lap, relieves you of the need to try to remember how many laps you have run.

I had quit using judo slippers after a few months because, running over a distance, they give no support to the arch and no cushion to protect the soles of the feet and they are useless for outdoor running. I experimented with a variety of running shoes before settling on a pair of very light Japanese-made marathon running shoes, with a nylon upper and a ripple sole. I still use them after having run through three pairs.

I made many mistakes in that first year, the most painful being a tendency to run the first mile too fast. I began doing that when I got the stopwatch, trying to break my personal record each time I ran, a manifest impossibility.

It would be hard to exaggerate the importance of an adequate warm-up period before running. When I began, I walked a couple of laps to warm up; later I started doing ten minutes of light calisthenics before going onto the track. Still later, after I had reached the three-mile plateau, I discovered that I could improve my times by running the first mile slowly, picking up the pace in the second, and running the third at what, for me, was a fairly hard pace.

At this time, I tried to keep a nine-minute mile or better pace, aiming for eight-minute miles on the days when I felt particularly good. By the end of the year, I was consistently under twenty-seven minutes for three miles, but I do not recommend anyone setting goals and if I were starting over again, I don't think I would buy a stopwatch.

As you begin to run more easily and faster, you have a lamentable tendency to think of yourself as an athlete and no man in his fifties is that. It can, very literally, be a fatal mistake. The heart and lungs benefit as much from a leisurely pace continued over a length of time as they do from a straining mile and the chance of taxing a weak heart beyond its ability to respond is much less.

Bill Bowerman, the track coach at the University of Oregon, has produced some of the great milers of recent track history, including Dyrol Burleson. In addition to coaching the university track team, Bowerman conducts classes in jogging for the middle-aged in the vicinity of Eugene, where the school is located.

I have known Bill for a long time and, after I had been running for some nine months, I ran into him at a track meet in California one afternoon.

I told him what I had been doing, expecting him to be impressed, but he was not.

"I'll tell you the same thing I tell my joggers," he said. "Train, don't strain. I tell them to jog at a pace easy enough for conversation, so that you can talk to someone while you're running. Take it easy. You're not training for competition, you're training to maintain fitness. If you make it hard work, it'll be a lot more difficult to keep going and it could kill you."

It is not easy to slow down, but it is wise. I think I finally learned that lesson from Bob Cooper, a small man who has very likely run more miles on the West Side Y track than anyone else in the entire history of the place.

Bob is an attorney who appears to be in his mid-fifties. I don't remember when I first became aware of him because for much of the first two or three months I ran at the Y, I was not aware of anything other than the difficulty I was having in drawing a deep enough breath.

I noticed him finally because he was always on the track when I began my stint and still on it when I finished. He went slowly enough; after the first couple of months I found myself passing him every six or eight laps, which was not always easy, since he usually trailed a comet's tail of two to five men, all of them using him as a pacesetter, none of them going the full distance with him.

After I bought the lap counter and the stopwatch, I kept my mind off the tedium of running by trying to keep track of how far and how fast the other runners on the track were going. After some fairly complicated mental arithmetic based on my own pace and how often I lapped Bob, I decided that he was doing eleven- to twelve-minute miles. I had no idea how many he was doing each day, but it was certainly quite a few more than my two or three.

Each day when I started running, usually at about one in the afternoon, Bob would be on the track, a towel around his neck and his gray sweat shirt already dark with sweat.

He used a short, neat, and economical stride and looked absolutely tireless. After I had reached a distance and a time I considered respectable, I introduced myself to him and asked him how far he ran each day.

"Six to nine," Bob said. "I used to do more than that, but I have had a problem with my legs in the last couple of years, so I had to cut down the pace and the distance. Maybe you've noticed that I stop now and then for a couple of minutes?"

I hadn't noticed, probably because he hadn't had to rest during the brief periods I spent on the track.

He had phlebitis, a disease which inhibits circulation, in his legs so that, after he had run a while, the muscles became tight and painful from lack of oxygen. I found out later that Bob had been a very good distance runner earlier.

"He ran in the marathon quite a few times," Crichton told me. "And damn well. He used to go with me when I was running well and I couldn't outrun him."

Bob would warm up for his daily run by riding the stationary bicycle for twenty or twenty-five miles first, and one afternoon I talked to him as he pedaled away.

"It must be tough to cut down on your speed so much," I said. At the time I was trying desperately to build my own pace, with some success.

"I used to feel that way," he said. "But I suppose the really important thing is to keep going, no matter how slow you run. I wish I could do seven-minute miles all day, the way I used to. But I enjoy running now and I have found out in the last few years that I enjoy it just as much without trying to break any records."

"Doesn't it bother you when the runners you used to lap, lap you?"

"No," Bob said. "Not really. More power to them. I get a kick out of watching them come on. I'd hate to have to count how many I've watched from the time they start, fat and timid and slow, until they reach the point where they lap me every five or six turns of the track. By that time, I know most of them and I enjoy watching their progress."

"How about your legs?" I asked. "Can't anything be done about the circulation?"

"Nothing has worked so far," he said philosophically. "It's something I have to live with. You have to run through the pain, you see. When it gets too bad, I stop for a while. But I've never even considered giving up running. It becomes an addiction after a while."

Jogging seemed more an affliction than an addiction to me then, but by the end of the year, I understood Cooper better. Running had not become an unalloyed pleasure to me, but it had become a necessity. I went the first year without missing a scheduled run and when I finally did miss one, I felt miserable.

I suppose it would be more accurate to say that running becomes an obsession after a time. The physical act of running gradually becomes less onerous and much less painful as you develop heart and lung capacity and the creaky ligaments in knees and ankles regain their flexibility, but I doubt that running itself is an actual pleasure for anyone.

In England, toward the end of my first year of jogging, I went to a track meet in which Ron Hill, the magnificent English distance runner, and Derek Clayton, the Australian marathoner, were competing. I talked with them after they had run, trying to find out how they reacted to the amazing amount of mileage they put in in preparation for their world record times.

"It's no lark," Hill said to me. "Running is never that, certainly. It's a bloody bore at best and damned painful at worst, but then I don't even approach Clayton's training schedule."

Clayton has run the fastest marathon in history, covering the 26 miles, 385 yards in an almost unbelievable two hours, eight minutes plus, which works out to a bit less than five minutes per mile. Since I knew very well that

I would be very lucky if I ever approached seven minutes for *one* mile, I looked at Clayton as if he were a superman, which indeed he is.

"He doesn't talk much about it," Hill said. "But I've trained with him in Australia. On my long day, I go up into the hills in the morning and run a twenty-seven-mile course, going a good pace and Derek runs with me. For me, that's the lot for the day. Derek goes back in the afternoon and runs another twenty."

"You must love to run," I said to Clayton. I could not conceive of anyone running forty-seven miles in a day without getting some pleasure from it.

"I hate it," Clayton said. "Absolutely. But I want very much to be the best in the world at something and I'll make the sacrifice for that."

I can't say that I found that very encouraging. Hill and Clayton were probably the two fittest runners in the world over distance and neither of them seemed to get any pleasure at all out of training. The pleasure came in competing and winning and I was far beyond competing and winning even in age-class races, in which runners of the same age race against one another.

I was still plagued, of course, by the bugaboo of competition and I had not yet reached the realization that for a middle-aged man recovering from a heart attack, running is a recreation, not a competition. That realization came over the next year.

Chapter Nine /

If the running itself is sometimes painful and often boring, the people you meet on the track and in the streets as you run compensate for much of it.

I spent a month in London in the early summer of 1969, staying at a flat in Chelsea. The London YMCA does not have an indoor track; there are no indoor tracks anywhere in England, for that matter, since the English are a hardy race who regard any temperature over seventy-five degrees as a heat wave. There are many more English joggers per capita than there are American and they go out to train in appalling weather, considering it bracing.

I wound up jogging at the Duke of York Headquarters on—or rather, *in*—the Kings Road in Chelsea. The Duke of York Headquarters is something like a National Guard armory in the States, albeit much more extensive and a bit more elaborate. The Home Forces use it for training and there is a running track, just off the Kings Road.

The track is an odd size, four and three-quarter laps to the mile, which makes for difficult arithmetic when you want to run three and a half, which I did on odd days. The infield is beautifully kept green lawn upon which small boys exercise in the early afternoon. The athletic grounds are kept up by a cheerful, wiry Englishman named Charlie Howells, who has been there for quite a few years. There have been some memorable English runners who trained at the Duke of York, but the performer Charlie remembers best is Prince Charles, who played cricket on the infield with his schoolmates. His old school still uses the training grounds for their recreation.

Our flat was only a few blocks from the track and at first I used to take my running gear with me in an airlines flight bag and change in the dressing room at the track, but I found rather quickly that the English do not believe in coddling their athletes.

The dressing room at the Duke of York was a small, bare room with wooden benches along the side and hooks in the wall for clothing. There was a toilet and two showers. The floor was cement and the heating was nonexistent. In early summer in England, the temperature sometimes hovers just above freezing, and it did just that for most of my stay.

After three or four days of shivering showers under a thin, lukewarm stream of water and a freezing ten minutes while I toweled frantically and dressed like a fireman, I decided that I would rather put up with the scorn of the English runners on hand than catch pneumonia. From then on, I walked to the track in a heavy nylon sweat suit, ran in it until I warmed up, then stripped to my running suit to finish, putting the sweat suit back on under a raincoat for the walk back to the apartment and a hot bath.

The Kings Road is one place where no one looks askance at your clothes, since the pedestrians there wear everything from a proper English suit to Levis and a T-shirt.

Once an elderly lady, who was standing with me waiting for a chance to cross the Kings Road, looked curiously at my blue nylon sweat suit and red running shoes.

"What kind of costume is that, sir?" she asked at last.

"It's a sweat suit, ma'am," I told her.

"A *sweat* suit?" she said doubtfully.

"Yes, ma'am," I said, wondering if I should try to explain.

"Coo," she said. "You Americans! Imagine wearing a proper costume just to perspire in!"

The Duke of York track was closed on Saturday and Sunday, so that on Saturday I had to find another place to run. I was a bit reluctant to trot through the streets of London in a nylon track suit, although I had seen plenty of English joggers doing their daily run through Hyde Park in shorts.

Although the English are much less given than Americans to shouting insults at joggers and other eccentrics, they are not perfect in that respect. Just after we arrived in London, the papers carried a story of an unhappy confrontation between a runner and a lorry driver.

The jogger was paddling along the street, presumably minding his own business, when the truck driver honked at him and yelled, "Knickers!"

Since knickers are ladies' panties in England, the jogger took understandable umbrage and challenged the truck driver. He wound up with a broken nose for his trouble and filed suit against his insulter. I don't know how the suit came out but, for the well-being of English joggers, I hope the lorry driver was taken off the streets for a while.

I solved the Saturday problem by running in the very early morning, before the lorries began rumbling through the streets of London. I worked out a three-miles-plus route which took me from the Kings Road over the Chelsea Bridge, through Battersea Park, back across the Thames on the Albert Bridge, then back to Kings Road.

I would run at about six in the morning, enjoying the cool, crisp feel of the London air before it had been polluted by engine exhausts. The streets would be all but empty, with only an occasional milk truck on its early rounds to disturb the peace. The few pedestrians abroad at the crack of dawn either greeted me cheerfully as I trotted by them or looked at me in quiet surprise.

The first time I made the run, after working out the route on a London street guide, I found my way easily enough until I had come back across the Thames on the Albert Bridge. Then I decided to detour through the small side streets between the Thames and the Kings Road and in about ten minutes I was completely lost.

I trotted along slowly, looking for a familiar street

name or a pub I might recognize, but the farther I went, the stranger the neighborhood seemed. I had been running almost forty-five minutes and, while I was not especially tired, I began to wonder how I would ever find my way back to the flat, since in the back streets no one was up and about.

Finally, as I reached the top of a small hill, I saw a bobby a half block away and trotted up to him, running in place when I stopped, and asked him where I could find the Kings Road.

He looked at me imperturbably, as if every Saturday morning in the gray light of the dawn, a gray-haired man in red shorts, a yellow singlet, and red track shoes, sweating profusely, jogged up to him for directions.

"Run to the bottom of the road, sir," he said politely, "then turn left."

He touched his cap in an informal salute and walked off without looking back.

In Mexico City, where I went to cover the world soccer championships, I again ran in the early hours of the morning; there was no track near my hotel, so I ran in Chapultepec Park, a beautiful, green place with winding roads and the Mexico City zoo. I ran through the zoo a few times, but the animals were usually asleep, except for the owls in the aviary.

The only other inhabitants of the park so early were neophyte matadors. There were two clearings in the woody sections of the park and both had been converted into makeshift bull rings, where ragged youngsters took turns passing a pair of bull's horns mounted on a bicycle wheel while a retired torero schooled them in the intricacies of the various passes.

I stopped a few times to watch them quietly and they paid little attention to me. I suppose that even horns mounted on a bicycle wheel and operated by another youngster can be dangerous if you don't concentrate.

There were problems running in Mexico City which did not exist in London. The first morning I ran there, I went out in my usual shorts and singlet and drew so many insults from passing Mexicans that for the next three weeks I ran in regular trousers and shirt.

Then the air in Mexico City is the most polluted in any major city in the world, with the possible exception of Tokyo. And to make it worse, Mexico City is 7,000 feet up, so that the air is thin and breathing much more difficult. By the time I went to Mexico City, I was up to from five to ten miles a day, but I found it impossible to go that far through the thin, polluted air. I cut my daily stint down to three miles and went appreciably slower than I had been running at sea level.

By the end of the three weeks of running at altitude, I had become a bit more acclimated, but I was never really comfortable. When I returned to New York and the familiar track at the Y, I found that the altitude work had made running a distance much easier.

One of the problems which creates a handicap in maintaining a jogging program and traveling widely at the same time is the physical stress of a major change in time zones.

The time difference between London and New York, for example, is five hours and it takes at least a week for the body metabolism to make the adjustment required to compensate for sleeping and eating at different times. Your body stays on New York time while you operate on London time and the result is that you go very flat, physically, for several days. I knew this from my experience with the United States track and field team in the Olympics in Rome in 1960.

I was covering the games and the United States, as usual, had sent what should have been easily the strongest team in the world to represent America.

One of my particular friends on the team was Jim Beatty, the little five-thousand-meter runner who was given a very strong chance to break the foreign monopoly which existed in distance running at the time. He had been running superbly in the United States before coming to Europe.

Shockingly, Jim did not even qualify for the finals in the five thousand. He ran some thirty seconds slower than his U.S. times. We had dinner the night after he had failed so signally.

"I thought I was fit," he told me miserably, fighting to hold back tears. "I had put the money in the bank. I never worked so hard in my life as I did for this chance and today I didn't have a thing. I tried, but I felt dead."

The same day, all three of the U.S. half-milers, rated among the top ten in the world, were eliminated in heats and all of them had had the same dull, flat feeling that Jim had.

Unfortunately for them, and for the United States, they had been forced to compete in the middle of the physical doldrums brought on by the major time change. The worst of the flat period comes a week or ten days after the time change, which coincided with the opening of the track and field competition. Although the effect on a jogger is not quite so drastic, it is certainly appreciable and there is nothing to do about it but wait for the body to make the adjustment.

The time change from New York to Los Angeles is three hours, but it does not seem to have nearly so severe an effect.

Chapter Ten /

When I began jogging, I had no idea how many other joggers I would run into during the course of the first year. One of the constants in running, no matter where I was, was the presence of other joggers, even in the dawn hours—in Chapultepec and London.

Fifteen years ago, there were only a few eccentrics who spent time trundling across the countryside in search of health and fitness; the most recent estimate of the number of joggers in the United States now is about ten million. My dentist in Manhattan starts his day by running three miles up and down the East River Drive; there were about eighty doctors who finished in the Boston Marathon in 1971.

In the spring of 1969, I did a story on jogging and got

an avalanche of mail from joggers all over the world.

The story began, strangely enough, at six in the morning in the Astrodome in Houston, Texas, with Judge Roy Hofheinz, the portly owner of the Houston Astros and most of the real estate surrounding the Astrodome, running a foot race from home plate to first base against Louie Welch, the mayor of Houston.

The judge weighs something more than 230 pounds and he had not run at all for years, so Mayor Welch won in a canter, despite the judge's spectacular uniform. He wore a sweat suit with "Here come da Judge" lettered on the front and "Dere go da Judge" on the back.

The reason for the race was a Jog-In, an event sponsored by two disc jockeys, Mack Hudson and Irving Harrigan, from radio station KILT. They had proposed the idea more or less as a gag but, surprisingly, 6,300 Houstonians appeared at the ungodly hour of six to trot three times around the baseball field in honor of jogging.

Judge Hofheinz, incidentally, took his defeat with reasonably good grace.

"That's the first time Louie has beaten me in three races," he said good-naturedly. "I guess he was due." The other races, the judge did not point out, had been political.

The starter for their historic match was Dr. Denton Cooley, the Houston surgeon who has performed more heart transplants than any other surgeon in the world. Cooley is himself a jogger, but he was on hand to petition donations of vital organs for the Living Bank, for eventual use in transplants. The organs, offered with surprising generosity by the joggers on hand, were for future delivery, of course.

The two disc jockeys who had started the whole thing were a bit bemused by the unexpected success it had.

"All we offered was a free sweat shirt," Hudson said. "Not even a sweat shirt, really, just a T-shirt. We had a couple of thousand of them, figuring that would be plenty and we ran out by six in the morning. It's amazing. I guess we'll have to do it every year."

Not long after the Jog-In at the Astrodome, I was in Long Beach, California, for another jogging celebration, this one a Witness to Fitness meeting sponsored by the Long Beach Community Hospital to dedicate thirty-four jogging trails that had been opened in the Long Beach area.

The jogging trails are on the grounds of fourteen public parks in the city, plus three high schools and thirteen junior highs, but I ran at the YMCA, after attending the opening ceremonies at the campus of California State College of Long Beach. I had been running for a year by then, but the spry elderly gentlemen who took part in a nine-mile jaunt beginning at eight in the morning shamed me into retiring to the Y indoor track.

There were some five hundred runners at this meeting, sixty of them doctors. Probably the most memorable was a tiny, muscular man named Fred Grace, whose face revealed his seventy-two years, but whose body looked a good thirty years younger. On that hot, sunny Saturday morning, Grace ran nine miles as easily as I might have run two, moving with a long, easy stride and showing no distress at all when he finished.

Nine miles, for Grace, was actually only a warm-up. Two years before, to celebrate his seventieth birthday,

Grace ran a hundred miles in three days, going a third of the distance each day nonstop.

I talked to him immediately after he had finished his running; he was breathing no harder than I was and all I had done was watch.

He laughed when I suggested that he must have been running all his life.

"No," he said. "Only about six or seven years. I was very active in judo until I was sixty-five and they said I was too old for strenuous exercise. So I took up running just to prove how wrong they were. I've been fit all my life and I do lots of repetition presses and squats with weights, but I've only been a serious runner lately."

He jogged away to warm down with a mile or two on the track. There were still runners on the oval, some of them women, a few children. Incredibly, a man who looked to be in his mid-twenties came by running on stumps. He had no feet and wore small, round pads over the stumps where his feet should have been. He was going at a good pace and I watched him for a long time.

"Amazing, isn't he?" someone said beside me and I turned to see a man in his mid-thirties. He was in running clothes and looked very fit, as did almost everyone there, with the possible exception of me.

"He was born without feet," he went on. "And only half a hand. But he has been running for years. You're actually looking at a medical impossibility. When I was in medical school, they told us that if a patient lost more than half a foot, he would never be able to walk normally, but he runs and runs well. Would you like to talk to him?"

I nodded and he stopped the footless runner, who walked over to me easily.

I felt a bit diffident about questioning him about his deformity, but he was cheerful enough about it and not at all reluctant to discuss it.

"I'm used to being stared at by now," he said, and smiled. "And I'm used to the questions, too. I know how strange it must seem to you, but I was born without feet, so I've never known anything else. I suppose if I had lost them in an accident, I would never have been able to walk, let alone run. But I guess running is just as natural to me as it is to you."

As he talked, he maintained his balance as easily as I did. He had a strong, lean body and well-developed muscles.

"There weren't really many sports I could go in for," he said matter-of-factly. "So I took up running."

Later, at a cocktail party for the sponsors and the press, I met a couple I had noticed during the morning. They had run the nine-mile course together, starting and finishing side by side.

The Jim Varelas are from Tustin, California, where he is a construction engineer. Jim is forty-seven and his wife, Isa, forty-five, and they celebrated their twentieth wedding anniversary by running twenty miles together.

"It wasn't bad," Isa said. "I got a little tired toward the end and I got blisters, but I wouldn't mind doing it again."

She stopped and giggled.

"Except for one thing," she said. "Jim had to stop a couple of times and go off into the woods for a couple of minutes and I knew if I stopped running, I would stiffen up and have a hard time starting again, so I ran around in circles while I waited for him. A lot of people looked at me as if I had lost my mind and one asked me what

I was doing, but I couldn't really tell him, could I?"

Isa is an exceptional runner for a woman and she carries over her extraordinary energy into promoting jogging for others. The last time I heard from her, she was busy trying to have an abandoned stretch of railroad track surfaced in asphalt so that it could be used for another running trail. I suspect that she'll be running on it before long.

But probably the most surprising of the female joggers is Super Sue Bailey, the pride of the Canton, Ohio, jogging set. Super Sue regularly does twenty miles a day and has done thirty-six without pause; when the Canton YMCA joggers set a national record by jogging 3,000 miles in four and a half days, Super Sue accounted for 208 of them, being exceeded only by two other joggers, both men.

Another jogging wife is Millie Cooper, wife of Dr. Kenneth Cooper, the Author of *Aerobics*, which might well be called the joggers' Bible. Dr. Cooper, a lean ex-miler from the University of Kansas, runs from four to six miles a day and Millie runs a mile and a half.

She accepted Dr. Cooper's jogging as just another husbandly eccentricity for a long time before she began running herself.

"After we got married, I didn't take any exercise," she told me. She is a very pretty brunette, almost as slim as her husband, who has the build of a whippet.

"I was getting fat and not doing anything about it," she went on. "I thought Kenneth was a nut. It never occurred to me that running would do me any good."

After the overwhelming success of Dr. Cooper's book, she tried jogging herself and has never stopped.

"One night, after the book was on the best-seller list, Kenneth looked at me and I guess there was quite a lot to look at," she said, and smiled.

"Millie," Dr. Cooper had said, "after all I said about overweight in the book, I can't afford to have a fat wife. You better start losing or looking."

"I think he was only kidding," Millie said doubtfully. "Anyway, I didn't start jogging for a while. He convinced me one night when we were sitting before the fireplace and he asked me to take his pulse."

Dr. Cooper, like all fit joggers, has a slow pulse because his heart pumps more blood per beat than the heart of a non-runner.

"I took his pulse and it was something like fifty-five beats a minute," Millie told me. "Then he took mine and it was going about eighty a minute. So he said, 'Millie, while we're sleeping tonight, your heart will beat about a third more times than mine and wear out about that much faster, too. How do you like that? When your heart has worn itself out, mine will still be going strong.'"

She paused a moment and felt her pulse, which is down near her husband's by now.

"I got to thinking about that," she said. "I mean, I thought about some other old girl coming in and taking over after I was gone and I didn't like it a little bit. I'm a very jealous girl and I started running the next day."

Chapter Eleven /

When I talked to Dr. Cooper for the *Sports Illustrated* jogging story, he lived in San Antonio, where he was a lieutenant colonel in charge of the United States Air Force Physical Fitness Program. He and Millie and Berkley, their three-year-old daughter, lived, fittingly, on Inspiration Drive and all three of them ran up and down the Inspiration Drive hill every evening.

Well, Berkley didn't really run. She's a bit young for that, although she is already a competitor.

"I run at least three miles in the morning, then I run a mile and a half with Millie when I get home," Dr. Cooper explained to me. "In order to make it fairer, I push Berkley in front of me in a stroller. And she gets mad if I fall behind. She likes to stay in front."

Cooper himself is a fine example of the advantages of the aerobic way of staying fit. He is forty years old and looks thirty, his body trim, all excess fat burned away on the road, his face looking almost drawn, the skin stretched tight over the bone structure. The leanness of the long-distance runner or jogger is of a different order from the leanness of the ordinary man.

A test to determine whether or not you are carrying any extra weight is the pinch test, taken on the stomach or the back of your upper arm. If, when you pinch the flesh there, you gather in a thickness of more than an inch of skin and fat, then you're overweight.

Cooper, in a test of this kind, would get only a double thickness of skin; he did not, however, achieve this spectacular degree of fitness in a couple of years; he has been running most of his life.

He was raised in Oklahoma and he ran the mile in 4:30.9 minutes for Putnam City High School before going to the University of Kansas, where his best time was a respectable 4:18.

"If I had trained really hard, I might have done better than that," he said. "But I was a premed and I actually did not have much time for training. We weren't doing the distances that milers put in today, but I wouldn't have been able to invest that much time, anyway."

I talked to him in his office at Lackland Air Force Base near San Antonio, a small, rather bare room, surprisingly unimpressive for a man with a job as important as Dr. Cooper's. He is a friendly, communicative man who gives you all his attention when he talks to you and who talks well and with a pleasant leavening of humor.

Aerobics, which has sold nearly three million copies in

hard cover and paperback, has made a dramatic change in the author's life. Dr. Cooper spends a great deal of time now lecturing; when I talked to him in San Antonio, he was doubtful about his future with the Air Force, because he was finding it difficult to get enough appropriations to implement his fitness program as fully as he would have liked.

He is, of course, a strong advocate of jogging as probably the best way to obtain maximum fitness results, although in his books, he has tables of values for almost any exercise you can imagine. Like most fitness experts, he does not think very highly of golf as an exercise.

"Golf is certainly better than nothing at all," he said in the tiny office. "But it does not create the training effect since it does not impose any real strain on the cardiovascular system."

"Golf," another famous doctor and heart specialist once said, "is a good way to spoil a walk." A walk, to have any aerobic effect, must be brisk and long enough to produce some degree of effort.

Although Dr. Cooper can cite many examples of men who have been helped by jogging, he is not universally admired by heart specialists, some of whom still retain the idea that anyone who has suffered a heart attack should spend the rest of his life avoiding exercise of any kind.

Indeed, there are some heart specialists who believe very strongly in the efficacy of exercise to rehabilitate a weakened heart who are still critical of Dr. Cooper.

One of them is Dr. Herman Hellerstein of Case Western Reserve University in Cleveland, Ohio. Dr. Hellerstein is an eminent specialist who has his own post-cardiac patients running up to two miles a day.

But he has a healthy suspicion of indiscriminate running.

In a panel discussion of exercise and post-cardiac care, he put it rather bluntly.

"I think competitive running is perfectly fine if the competitors are properly evaluated, properly trained, and properly supervised," he said. "All of life is competitive and I am for it. . . . I think it enhances survival, but it has to be done under the proper conditions. . . . I am not for the indiscriminate, unsupervised, unmonitored, self-prescribed competitive jogging, and you see pictures of Ken Cooper in every newspaper leading a pack of rats running down the public squares."

Cooper has not been pictured quite that often, either running alone or as a modern Pied Piper of Hamelin. There have been pictures of him running with his wife and daughter, which Millie dislikes almost as much as Dr. Hellerstein, since she feels that she looks a bit too wide in them, which she does not.

"None of these people have been evaluated," Dr. Hellerstein went on, speaking of the pack of rats supposedly led by Dr. Cooper. "I am against that and I have told Dr. Cooper that directly. . . . In the way of all flesh, it is not how far you go but how fast you try to get there . . . not too fast, not too slow, just right. Now this philosophy, applied to doctors, patients, businessmen, lawyers, what have you would be good."

When I quoted Dr. Hellerstein to Dr. Cooper in the small office in San Antonio, he smiled faintly, then grimaced.

"Dr. Hellerstein is a brilliant man," he said. "He has

done some wonderful things. I have heard that before and of course, I do *not* believe in any unsupervised exercise, not even for the young men who come here as Air Force cadets."

He got up from behind his small desk and stretched restlessly. He is not a man who takes kindly to sitting still for a long time; even seated, he seemed poised for action.

"The worst thing you can do is force yourself too hard," he said. He looked at me and frowned. "No man who has been sitting still for twenty years can go out and run hard. You have to start very easily. You should warm up for five or ten minutes before you start and cool down for at least that long when you finish."

I had told him about my own modest three miles a day and I was not sure that he wasn't warning me that I was doing too much, so I asked him if he thought I should cut back.

"No," he said quickly. "Not if it doesn't tax you too much. But I don't think you have to do any more than that."

He sat down again and watched disapprovingly as I lit a cigarette. I had gone over two hours without smoking one, trying to avoid smoking in front of him, but that was about my limit.

"There haven't been many fatalities from running," he said, "but the few there have been have all come— more or less—from the same things. An unconditioned man goes out and runs hard or he runs without a warm-up and finishes and walks directly to his car, without walking a while to warm down, and sits down behind the wheel.

"When you run hard for a long time, something like sixty percent of the blood in your body pools in your legs. If you quit running all at once and sit down, it remains in your legs, and it is almost impossible for the blood to get back up to your heart and brain. Because you are suffering from a deficiency of blood in your brain, you may faint."

I thought to myself how fortunate I had been not to have run under just that set of circumstances. I had always warmed up before running, but when I finished, I headed for my locker or my hotel room and did not bother warming down. Luckily, I had to walk down two flights of stairs at the Y and always a considerable distance to my car or my hotel room when I ran outdoors, so that I warmed down without realizing it.

"If you are standing up and faint," Dr. Cooper went on, "you fall down and the blood can get to your brain without fighting gravity so you come to rather quickly. If you walk over to your car and sit down behind the wheel and faint, the wheel holds you upright so that the blood cannot get back to your head or your heart and you can die. The autopsy won't show any heart damage, but you will die."

There have, of course, been heartening experiments by cardiologists in rehabilitating heart patients with jogging; Dr. Hellerstein in Cleveland, who decried Dr. Cooper's aerobic program, has a program with post-cardiac patients in which he gets his patients up to two miles a day and he has significantly reduced their mortality rate over the crucial five years subsequent to the attack. Dr. Viktor Gottheimer, in Tel Aviv, has established an even more remarkable record and reduced the mortality rate even further by training his post-cardiac patients to the point where they run *six* miles a day.

Many cardiologists believe wholeheartedly in the efficacy of running both to prevent and to heal heart attacks. But the medical profession moves very slowly in accepting new theories.

Very few people who die of heart attacks actually die while running or exercising. By far the most die in bed, or some time after having exercised. Of course, when you consider the statistics involving the amount of time people spend jogging and the amount they spend in bed, it is perfectly obvious that most people will die in the bed.

But there are rare cases of joggers dying while jogging and there is no medically accepted proof that jogging has lengthened anyone's life. There are thousands of people like me who believe wholeheartedly that jogging has, indeed, contributed to a more vigorous and probably a longer life, but there has so far been no accepted long-range study involving enough subjects and a blind control that proves this.

In early 1971, an anonymous doctor who is himself a jogger wrote a piece for a magazine called *Fitness for Living*, in which he cited the death of a jogger while jogging.

Because the article is written by a doctor who lost a friend who was also a doctor, it has particular cogency for anyone who, like myself, has had a heart attack and is running. It is worth reproducing here almost in its entirety for the cool intelligence with which the anonymous author examines the pros and cons of exercise and the heart. It begins:

He was 43, but he didn't look it. He could have claimed 38 and no one would have argued the point. He was robust and healthy and vivacious, a truly remarkable achiever in the prime of life. Some two months previously he had successfully passed a thorough physical examination.

For 17 years he had been my partner in the practice of medicine, for some eight years my partner, almost daily, in jogging and tennis. Then one day about dusk, just a few weeks ago, with about 1½ miles of his jogging route behind him and about a half mile to go, he fell in his tracks. Twenty minutes later, in the emergency room of the hospital he had founded, he was pronounced dead on arrival.

Such was the shock of his death to the community that the phone calls, loaded with questions about jogging—the why of it, the wisdom of it—are still coming in. In the wake of such tragedy, some 'mental jogging' has become very much in order.

Sudden, unexpected death among physical fitness enthusiasts is nothing new, and although by no means common, it is, by the same token, far from rare. When a person reads of it in a total stranger, he shakes his head, makes a mental note of it, and passes on. But when it strikes down one as close as a brother, a medical partner of almost two decades, one whose jogging steps he has heard alongside his own year after year after year, he calls a halt—takes time out for an inventory.

One asks, under such circumstances, what about physical fitness, really? Is it everything it's cracked up to be? Do its benefits really outweigh the risks involved? And jogging, in particular—that highly touted, superlative form of fitness endeavor—is it in reality a wolf in sheep's clothing?

After my long-time companion and friend went down, all alone, in a park behind his home, I asked myself these questions—and many more. To some such questions the answers are crystal clear. To others, more time and further research is needed.

For example, whether or not arduous leisure-time activity such as jogging is really an extender of life is still a moot question. Preliminary reports seem positive. Some statistics indicate that the chances of sudden unexpected death occurring during such sedentary activities as sitting or sleeping are on the order of 20 to 25 times greater than the chances of its occurring during vigorous activity.

That a good fitness program makes one "feel better" is open to little doubt. [If the good doctor needs another witness to this, I am available.] My stricken friend, and scores of others who have written or with whom I have talked, have all experienced that good feeling. But there still is no proof that leisure-time fitness programs extend life. What is known thus far is favorable, and if I had to gamble on the outcome of the statistics now being gathered, I'd put my money on well-tailored and sensibly managed physical fitness programs.

But I'm biased, I suppose, for I'm convinced that the credits of exercise far outweigh its debits, even if it is never shown to extend one's life a single day. I knew, for example, as my friend and I often discussed, if fitness did nothing else for us, it afforded excellent outlets for tension, a factor which I believe is the "fire under the pot" of fatty diets and inactivity and a dozen or more other environmental factors which make up the way of life fostering coronary heart disease.

I can see and hear my friend quite vividly even now as he would stroke a potent forehand shot across the net at me while yelling: "Just think! A psychiatrist would charge you $25.00 an hour for this!" How often we agreed that our midday break for tennis or jogging, considering the tensions it shed, ought to cost something more than an hour or so of time!

And then there's the diet thing. Each of us found it so much easier to control our weight and yet eat as much, calorically, as we wanted. Cholesterol levels declined as well.

Was the heart attack in some way related to his active life style? As it turned out, there was postmortem evidence that my friend had extensive atherosclerotic involvement of all his coronary arteries, a process that had been going on for decades in him. There was even evidence of old, though mute, heart attacks. [A mute heart attack is one you do not feel.] While it's easy to say that but for his fitness program he might be here today, I know it is equally possible that a heart attack might have cut him down years ago had he not been a regular participant in fitness.

Who can say?

Physical fitness, when all is said and done, is a way of life on which one must be sold by his or her own self, or it is no good. The fanatical devotion of its believers defies explanation. Like a religious encounter, it must be experienced. Mere words cannot explain it or do it justice. Nor can simply "tasting" it by way of one or two brief encounters. . . .

My friend's death has caused a lot of introspection—make no mistake—and brought on a barrage of such personalized questions as: "What are you going to do now? What do you think of fitness now?"

For what it's worth, here, very simply, is my answer: "I'll keep on running." And if the shoe were on the other foot, with my friend being here instead of me, I am equally confident that he would do the same.

Let's face it. No fitness program is entirely without risk, especially in those aged forty and over. But, for that matter, neither is any medication—and exercise is a form of therapy—completely hazard-free. A simple aspirin tablet may do you in. However, in the wake of such events, certain basics need to be reiterated once again. Here are some "mental jogs" for joggers that each would do well to keep in mind.

[The rules which follow are so basic and so generally advocated by *all* doctors who are conversant with the effects of exercise on the heart that I think any jogger, of any age, would be well-advised to copy them and reread them at regular intervals.]

(These recommendations were thoroughly reviewed and approved by Dr. Kenneth H. Cooper, author of *Aerobics* and probably the most renowned authority on physical fitness in America today.)

1. Unless under 35 years of age, without a history of serious illness at any time, no fitness program should be undertaken without prior thorough medical examination and expert advice. Such examinations must include some acceptable form of stress testing—i.e., monitoring the heart performance while the patient is engaged in physical activity. And, of course, they should be conducted by physicians well trained in exercise physiology. Oddly enough, very few general practitioners have the time or the knowledge to give meaningful exercise stress tests. Some physicians and exercise physiologists have formed teams and opened special labs to test people and write exercise prescriptions for them. (For help in contacting such a physician, or the labs, write *Fitness for Living*, Dept. L, Emmaus, Pa. 18049.)

2. Never attempt to "get in shape" overnight. Conditioning takes time. A number of good books, notably *The New Aerobics* (Kenneth Cooper, M.D.), are available as guides.

3. Get periodic monitored stress tests, (the older one is, the more frequently) preferably by physicians familiar with stress testing.

4. Even in the well-conditioned person, highly competitive participation in any sport should be evaluated thoroughly by a physician. *This includes running against the clock*—i.e., attempting to improve track performance.

5. If over age 35, or certainly 40, running (or similar activity) alone should be avoided if possible. Run in groups, or at least with someone who is familiar with resuscitative measures. Resuscitation must begin in the event of heart stoppage, within four minutes at the very most. Otherwise, even if recovery occurs, brain damage may result.

6. Always make allowance for such variables as heat, humidity, fatigue, recent illness, and stress.

7. After forced layoffs from a physical fitness program—as with illness—do not attempt to perform immediately at pre-layoff levels. Rather, first undergo slow and gradual reconditioning.

8. Preceding each session, warm up gradually and, following each exercise session, cool off gradually.

9. With the appearance of pain in or about the chest, arms, neck, head, ears, or upper abdomen, in particular, or in case of dizziness or undue shortness of breath, stop activity at once and report to your physician.

10. Do not eat a heavy meal within two (or preferably three) hours of an exercise session.

Yes, I have lost a good friend, an irreplaceable partner, and a fellow fitness enthusiast, but, as I have said, I shall do exactly what my friend would do were the situation reversed. I'll keep on running. After all, with odds like 20 to 1, a guy has to run pretty hard to keep from dying in bed. Don't you agree?

Chapter Twelve /

No middle-aged man should run "hard." I made that mistake myself during my first year of jogging; recently I have quit using a stopwatch to record my times and made sure that I never tax myself to exhaustion. I reached a point where I could run a mile in seven minutes, but that should not be the goal of any jogger, whatever speed he is capable of.

Of course, the farther you run each day on a controlled program, the more fit you become, up to a point. When you go beyond that point and are still tired from the previous day's effort when you start to run, then you are running too far, obviously, and the time has come to cut back.

One of the more remarkable men I met in my pursuit

of information on the benefits of jogging is Seymour Lieberman, an attorney who lives in Houston, Texas.

Lieberman was very probably the first man in the country who dedicated himself to popularizing jogging as a means for fitness. I remember the first time I met him, in the late 1950s, in a small hotel room in Chicago. I was there to cover a track meet and Seymour, who is active in track and field, was there as an official.

He had asked me to come to his room to demonstrate to me the Seymour Lieberman plan for physical fitness, which he was trying to sell to the administration in Washington, with little success.

He is a small, intense man and at the time I thought that he was a bit ridiculous, although in retrospect, I have often wished I had taken the advice he gave me that day and paid closer attention to what he had to say.

He spent about an hour that day, jogging gently around the narrow confines of the hotel room, trying to sell me on doing a story and trying to interest a representative of President Kennedy's Council on Youth Fitness in sponsoring his ideas.

Ten years later, when I was working on the jogging story for my magazine, Lieberman was an obvious source, so I took the opportunity to talk to him while I was in Houston on another track story, the first indoor track meet in the Astrodome.

I was still fighting the battle of the stopwatch then and I looked forward to running on the huge, $60,000, five-laps-to-the-mile track that had been built for the meet.

I had an understandable reluctance to do my three miles on the track while the competitors were warming up, so I went to the Astrodome at eight in the morning of the first day of the meet. Workmen were installing the last sections to complete the oval, so that I had to run part of the time in the infield.

The workmen finished after I had run about a mile and the foreman stopped me as I came around. I thought for a moment that he was going to ask me to get off the track, although I had obtained special permission from the judge to use it, but he said, "How is the track?"

"Fine," I said, trying to appear a veteran of track meets. "Maybe a little soft on the curves, but very good."

"Thank you," he said respectfully and I jogged off feeling very athletic.

The feeling lasted only a couple more laps. By that time, a couple of dozen real athletes had arrived to warm up for morning heats and were zipping by me regularly, most of them looking back in amazement as they went by. By the time I had finished the three miles, a good deal faster than I had ever run three miles before, I was exhausted and the runners in the distance races must have been the most confident group ever to compete in a meet anywhere.

The next day, there were no morning heats and I had the track all to myself until a tour group filed into the stands and sat at one end, watching solemnly as I toiled around lap after lap. A small boy waved at me once and I waved back. The second time I went by, I heard him say, "But, Mama, he's so *old*." I agreed with W. C. Fields for the next couple of laps. He once said, "No one who hates dogs and children can be all bad."

I told Seymour about running in the Astrodome and told him my time for the three miles the first day, since I was rather proud of it.

He shook his head at me and said, "Throw away the watch. What you're doing is making jogging hard work. You're not going to be in the Olympics and you'll reach a limit to how fast you can go before long. When that happens, it may be so discouraging to you that you will quit running altogether."

It took quite a while for me to realize that Lieberman was right, but when I did, jogging changed from a painful chore to be performed every day into something approaching pleasure.

Seymour himself is a very strong runner, although he is in his sixties. As a high school senior, he tied the then world record for the fifty-yard dash (5.2) and went on to compete for Chicago's Loyola University.

He kept fit even after he had earned a law degree, and competed in walking races until he was thirty-six. By then, so much of his time was taken up by his burgeoning practice that he had to give up walking and confined his exercise to a very occasional round of golf.

"In the next nine years, I gained about fifteen pounds," he told me. "I wasn't fat by any means, but I was well over my fit weight. Then I began reading more and more often in the papers the obituaries of friends of my age—forty-five—who had died of a heart attack or of a stroke.

"I tried to figure out the best way to get myself back into condition, and I spent three months in research and analysis of various kinds of exercise. I came to the conclusion that the most efficient conditioning came from running. If a heavyweight fighter is training to go fifteen rounds, he runs at least five miles a day for endurance and condition. The work he does in the gymnasium is just to sharpen his coordination and his punching.

"I figured that slow running was the best way to put the body in good shape, so I started running. I went to my doctor every week for a checkup while I was doing it, because at that time, back in 1953, no one my age was running."

When he began jogging, Lieberman suffered from a sacroiliac pain. After six months of carefully supervised running, Lieberman discovered that his pulse rate had slowed appreciably, that his heart returned to normal much more quickly after exercise and that he no longer had the pain in his back.

"I came to the conclusion that I had been carrying four or five extra inches of fat on my belly," he said. "That threw me out of balance and put an unnatural strain on my back and caused the pain in the sacroiliac. I developed a habit of twisting my torso as I jogged, which helped take off the fat."

He got up from his desk and jogged in place for a few minutes, twisting his upper body from side to side, to demonstrate what he meant.

"I wear the same riding pants today that I wore twenty-seven years ago," he said when he had sat down again. "The fit is perfect."

As a demonstration of his fitness on his sixtieth birthday, Seymour arose early and ran three miles along the beach at Galveston, a much more difficult feat than running on a hard surface since the sand makes the going much harder. He then repaired to a nearby golf course and played eighteen holes, after which he went home to drink a glass of honey and lemon juice and rest for an hour.

After the rest, he swam a mile in the Gulf of Mexico, dressed, and drank some more honey and lemon juice, and went for a ten-mile ride on horseback.

"I was tired when it was over, but not unpleasantly so," he said. "I never exercise to exhaustion."

Lieberman never misses a scheduled workout and he has gone to rather unusual lengths to avoid it. When he was fifty-six, he caught pneumonia and was confined to hospital. When he is unable to run outdoors, he jogs in place as a substitute and during the three weeks he was confined, with temperatures ranging up to 102°, he jogged.

"My doctor was dubious about it," he said, "but I got out of bed and jogged in place for five minutes every day, which was quite a shock for my nurses. However, when I got up again at the end of the three weeks, I was ready to go back to work immediately, instead of having to be convalescent for three more weeks at home, as is usually the case after an attack of pneumonia."

Certainly no doctor in his right mind would recommend such heroics for the average patient, but then Seymour was not the average patient. Among his most prized possessions is a certificate from the International Council of Sport and Physical Education acknowledging that he is the founder of the jogging movement.

The third man, along with Dr. Cooper and Lieberman, who has been a major factor in the rising popularity of jogging is Bill Bowerman, the track coach at the University of Oregon in Eugene.

I had known Bowerman as one of the finest track coaches in the world for a long time before I became aware of his interest in jogging. He wrote a book called

Jogging, which I read even before I read Dr. Cooper's book. Since he has developed some of the greatest distance runners in track history, I read the book with a great deal of interest, then discussed jogging with Bill at a track meet on the West Coast.

"You would think that I'd have been jogging for a long time," Bill said, rather ruefully. He is a man about my age (middle fifties) and he has always looked very fit and strong. The only change I had noticed in him after not seeing him for a few years was that he was much leaner.

"I always thought that I was in pretty good shape," Bill went on. "I do a lot of walking and hunting and fishing, but I hadn't done any jogging until I went to New Zealand several years ago to talk to Arthur Lydiard."

Lydiard is the coach who trained Peter Snell, the Olympic 800-meter champion in 1960, among a host of other fine distance runners. He is a compact, leathery-looking man who runs only a little slower and little less than his runners.

"Lydiard asked me if I would like to go out with him for an early run," Bowerman said, and smiled. "So I went out and followed him for a while, trotting along easily enough. But we kept on trotting and trotting and trotting and by the time we went by six miles my tongue was hanging out and I was ready to cash in. Then we hit the hills."

(Hills are of tremendous importance in training competitive distance runners and they afford a pleasant view of the countryside for joggers, but most of them should be walked, not run.)

"By now I was barely walking," Bill recalled. "An

eighty-year-old man came jogging by me and said 'Come on, laddie, you're flagging.' "

Inspired by Lydiard and by the elderly runner, Bowerman began his own jogging program upon his return to Eugene. He also recruited a large group of other middle-aged men who take part in what may be the most extensive community jogging program in the country. His book, written in collaboration with Dr. Waldo Harris, preaches moderation and his program aims for a thirty-minute three miles.

Bowerman agrees with Lieberman and Dr. Cooper and indeed almost all advocates of jogging for health in the necessity for avoiding strenuous effort.

"I tell my joggers to run slowly enough so that they can talk while they jog," he says. "And, of course, it is literally true that you should walk before you run."

If all the strictures against really hard running are applicable to runners over thirty who have never had a heart attack, they are trebly applicable to middle-aged post-cardiac patients, such as I am. In my research on jogging, I have been very anxious to learn of other post-cardiac joggers and there are a few.

Dr. George A. Sheehan is a fifty-two-year-old cardiologist who lives in New Jersey and who was, in his youth, a sprinter for Manhattan College. In his youthful middle age, he is a distance runner who takes part in the Boston Marathon each spring and runs well enough to finish among the first two or three hundred out of the thousand or so competitors who show up each year.

He is a firm believer in jogging for the rehabilitation of victims of heart attacks. Recently, at a symposium on heart disease at a New York YMCA, he said, "Running not only improves a person's heart-lung capacity, but it translates heart disease prevention into a life style, an improved self-image, a philosophy that the body reflects the mind and soul."

At the same symposium, Rene Biourd, the physical director for the Grand Central YMCA in New York, reported on the results of a running class for sixty-five patients conducted at his Y over the past five years.

"There was only one heart relapse," he said. "The man who had it was pushing seventy and he was back on the track in two weeks."

In emphasizing the importance of running well within your physical abilities, Sheehan repeated what Lieberman had said.

"Throw away your stopwatch," he said. "Run at your own pace just for the pleasure of hearing your own healthy heartbeat." He feels that three exercise sessions a week, comprising aerobic warm-up, calisthenics, and fifteen or thirty minutes of jogging are enough to leave a post-cardiac patient in a glow of good, if not robust, health.

He took strong issue with President Nixon, who had, just before the symposium, said to the members of his Sports Advisory Council, "I really hate exercise for exercise's sake." He went on to add that he belonged to the beer-and-pretzel fans who prop their feet up in front of their TV sets for a long weekend of sportswatching, without physical participation of any kind.

"It's no disgrace if some people prefer their exercise vicariously," the President said. However, another story about the President revealed that he jogs in place for 400 steps every morning, which is hardly enough to have much effect on his fitness one way or the other.

"No wonder we have the highest heart attack rate in the world," Dr. Sheehan said in disgust after reading the President's comment. "Businessmen won't exercise at noon because of a shower hangup. They don't want to sweat. They're afraid of perspiration. What's wrong with a little honest sweat? If everybody ran, nobody would notice."

As more and more cardiologists come around to Dr. Sheehan's way of thinking, more statistics will be available on the survival rate of exercising post-cardiac patients as compared with the survival of less energetic patients.

The results obtained by the two most prominent experts on the rehabilitation of heart patients by exercise are Dr. Cooper's severest critics, Cleveland's Dr. Herman Hellerstein and Dr. Viktor Gottheimer of Tel Aviv.

Dr. Cooper, who bears no grudge against Hellerstein, has analyzed their results.

"In cases of heart attack," he said, "about fourteen percent of all victims die before getting to hospitals. Another nineteen percent die within the first four weeks. Of the survivors, twenty to twenty-five in a hundred usually die of another heart attack within five years."

These statistics do not hold, however, for the patients under the care of Drs. Hellerstein and Gottheimer.

"Dr. Hellerstein has, by carefully supervised exercise, cut the death rate from twenty-five in one hundred to fewer than ten in one hundred," Dr. Cooper says. "Dr. Gottheimer, who gradually brings his patients up to running as many as six miles a day, has done even better than that. He reports their mortality rate has fallen to fewer than five per hundred in the first five years subsequent to their attack, or five times less than patients who do not exercise."

Chapter Thirteen /

I finished my first full year as a jogger on September 1, 1969, leaner, faster, stronger, and, oddly enough, happier. One of the benefits of jogging, aside from the purely physical, is psychological.

Although jogging is not an unalloyed pleasure, it *does* have a very pleasant side effect. I can't think of anything which relaxes you more mentally or eases tensions more completely than a leisurely run. While you are running, you do not worry about anything. It is an all-absorbing occupation and when you have finished, the pleasant fatigue combined with the sense of accomplishment keeps tension away for a long time.

By the end of that first year, I was running three miles a day, five days a week. I had covered 713½ miles in 105 hours, 17 minutes, 4.2 seconds, adding distance and speed at an accelerating pace during the final six months. Once or twice, I ran four miles instead of three, but my regular schedule called for fifteen miles a week.

I had lost over forty pounds and seven inches from my waist and I felt better than I had for years, including most of the years before the heart attack. I had reduced my two-mile time by more than eight and a half minutes, time for a mile by almost five and I had too much ambition.

I started the second year by increasing my running stint from three to three and a half miles, five times a week, and set myself some fairly unrealistic goals, despite all the good advice I had had about discarding my stopwatch.

I decided that I would try for a six-minute mile, two miles in thirteen minutes and three in twenty-one, all performances which would be routine for a junior high school student but not for a heart patient.

For the first seven running days, I did the three and a half easily enough, then stepped it up to five miles on the eighth day and did the five handily. I called my wife from the Y to tell her I would be home a little later than I thought.

"I got carried away and ran five miles," I said.

"Keep that up and you will be," she said.

I ran five again a week later, followed by two fours; someone had once told me that after you reached the three-mile plateau, adding distance was no real problem and I found this to be true. I was really no more tired after jogging five miles than I had been after three and my pace was not that much slower.

Then, starting the fourth week of the second year, I ran into two problems that had bothered me intermittently during the first, but not enough to keep me from running.

I had a severe attack of gall bladder pain the night before my first running day in the fourth week, but I had had that before and run anyway and I did again. By morning, the gall bladder did not bother me, but when I ran, my right knee and thigh were painful, although I finished the three and a half miles in fairly good time.

By the time I had finished showering and started to dress, my right leg was so stiff that I had trouble getting my shoe on. The knee was swollen and red and very sore to the touch; once before, I had had a similar pain in my right big toe, before I had begun running, and the team doctor for the Green Bay Packers diagnosed it as gout.

The diagnosis for the knee was the same and the next day I began taking Benemid and Indocin, pills designed to lower the uric acid content of the blood. The pain of gout is caused by uric acid crystals that form in the joints; it is a rather cold comfort when you're suffering an attack to reflect that some researchers have discovered that high uric acid levels go along with high achievement and an unusual degree of intelligence.

The gout kept me off the track for a full week; later, when I felt twinges in my big toe, ankle, or knee, I knew enough *not* to run; in the early stages of gout, at least for me, the pain subsides after you have run a few laps but the running inflames the joint and makes the attack more severe than need be. I now take a pill that controls the uric acid level and I haven't had an attack of gout for a long time. I have an occasional twinge and I suppose I always will have, but rest and treatment usually clear it up in a couple of days so that my jogging program is not seriously hampered.

Gout can attack in any joint and often follows a slight injury; over the years, I have had it in my right big toe, ankle, and knee and left big toe and knee. There is no question of running when it is at its height; the pain in the joint is so severe that even the weight of a sheet becomes unbearable.

After the week's layoff necessitated by the gout, I cut back to two miles a day for five days, running rather slowly. The last two days, I ran at a golf course in San Diego, behind the motel where I was staying, going out at six-thirty in the morning each day and running through the dew still on the grass. The clean air and the quiet empty course made the running very pleasant. I have found golf courses ideal tracks in the early morning; later they become dangerous.

Herb Elliott, the Australian miler who won the 1960 Olympics by about as wide a margin as anyone ever won a world class 1,500-meter race, taught me about golf courses. In 1959, the year before the Olympics, I did a piece on Elliott and at one point drove him from Los Angeles to Compton, California, for a meet. The drive took two days and Herb went looking for a place to run after we had checked into our motel at the end of the first day.

The motel was called the Golden Tee and adjacent to it was a golf course. I asked the pro if it would be all right for Herb to run around the course two or three times and he nodded.

"Two or three times?" he said. "This course is a little

over 7,000 yards. That's well over three miles."

Herb ran the course twice; he was favoring a slight muscle pull in his calf and he didn't want to strain it. The late golfers, finishing their rounds in the gathering dusk, looked up in surprise as he loped by, but Herb ignored them. The next morning, we played the course together; Herb ran it much more easily than he played it.

Three days later, he had to drop out of the mile in the Compton meet; the muscle pull had not responded to rest and heat treatment.

I was luckier with the gout, but tnen I wasn't going fast enough to strain any muscles. When I returned to New York from San Diego, I increased my mileage to four miles a day and found that after five days, although I was a bit more tired than usual, I was not uncomfortably so and after a two-day rest, I was fresh and strong.

The next week, I varied the distances, starting with two miles, then running six the second day (the longest run I had made up until then) and following with five, four, and three. The five-mile run was a new personal record, under forty-five minutes, averaging less than nine minutes per mile. By now I had reached the point that Crichton once told me I would; the next week, intending to run five miles, I found, in the fifth mile, that I was not concious at all of laboring for my breath. I was breathing easily and hardly any harder than I would have been at a fast walk six months before, so I ran seven miles instead of five.

In the next few months, I found that the strong base of conditioning that I had built over the previous year made the distance I ran almost of no importance; one week I ran ten miles three days in a row and ran it faster the third day than I had the first. I had, running at my own speed, which was around nine minutes per mile, an almost inexhaustible capacity for endurance; the ten-mile runs lasted about an hour and a half each and I ran in the morning before going to my office.

Instead of feeling tired, I felt more alive and alert than I had for years. My wife and some of my friends—the non-runners—thought that I was too thin and too gaunt. But Jerry approved and the runners knew that I was in good shape.

On March 21, 1970, I observed the fourth anniversary of my massive heart attack by running twelve miles on the twenty-four-laps-to-the-mile track at the West Side Y. The day was overcast, with the temperature in the middle forties, an ideal day for running since the air was reasonably clean and it was cool enough to be invigorating.

I began running at six minutes after noon and finished a little less than two hours later. I had had a belated birthday party the night before and drunk more than I intended. I had smoked about a pack of cigarettes that day, but I did not smoke at all before running.

My notes on that day show that I woke up at 7 A.M., had a breakfast of scrambled eggs, bacon, grapefruit juice, and coffee, then went back to bed and napped until ten-thirty. I took 600 units of vitamin E, plus multivitamin, multimineral B-12 complex, vitamin A, C, D, and bone meal before I left for the track. That night, I took another 600 units of vitamin E.

I would like to put in an aside here about vitamin E, a vitamin about which very little is known in the United States. There has been no minimal daily requirement established for humans; indeed, most doctors maintain that we get all the vitamins of any kind that we need if we eat a reasonably balanced diet.

I had grown aware of vitamin E after reading a book called *Vitamin E: Your Key to a Healthy Heart* by Herbert Bailey. Much of the book was based on research by Dr. E. V. Chute, a Canadian heart specialist, who had had extraordinary success in rehabilitating heart patients with massive doses of vitamin E.

I did not feel especially fresh when I began the twelve-mile run, and I wrote in my notes that my legs were rather dead for the whole run, but my breathing was easy and no problem at all, even during the last two miles, when I picked up the pace markedly. "Finished with a fairly good sprint over the final seven laps," I wrote. "Felt tired at the end, but not as tired as I have been after some ten-mile runs. My legs were sore in the shower, but my recovery was very quick and by evening, I felt as good as new. Maybe I should begin to think about the marathon!"

The next day, I ran six miles and felt as if it were a sprint. One of the advantages of doing a fairly substantial run once or twice a week is that the five- and six-mile runs seem short.

I broke my personal record for six miles, too, averaging a little less than eight minutes and fifty seconds a mile. For the next few months, the running grew easier and easier and distances seemed shorter and the note I had made about the marathon, as a joke, began to seem a real possibility to me.

Among the beneficial effects of vitamin E on heart patients is its faculty for inhibiting clotting, so that the likelihood of an embolism is reduced. It also improves the ability of the blood to carry oxygen to the muscles, so that a smaller volume of blood carries an adequate supply. According to Dr. Chute, it also regulates the heart to a degree. All of the effects are not only useful to post-cardiac patients, but to anyone who exercises. Among the patients treated by advocates of vitamin E, oddly enough, have been race horses which produced better times after vitamin E than before.

In my own case, it is difficult to say what effect the massive doses have had, except that my performances have improved and I no longer take coumadin, the usual blood thinner recommended for post-cardiac patients.

Much of the vitamin E we might normally get from our daily diet is destroyed by modern methods of processing food, (the best source is wheat germ, destroyed in making white flour) so that when Dr. Chute maintains that almost everyone in the United States and Canada suffers from a deficiency of it, he may well be right. At any rate, no doctor has ever proved that massive doses of the vitamin have any deleterious effect of any kind. I myself believe that they do improve the efficiency of the heart and the ability of the blood to carry oxygen.

Certainly when, for one reason or another, I am not able to take the 1,200 units a day that seems to be right for me, I find running more difficult. That, of course, may be psychological, but for whatever reason, I find running easier on a heavy regimen of E. Since there is no medical advice on just how much E to take, I arrived at 1,200 units from reading Dr. Chute's book.

I would probably find it much, much easier if I could quit smoking and drinking, but I have not been able to do so and I suppose that I will also continue to smoke and drink in the future, to my detriment.

But I believe very firmly that regular jogging also cuts down on the harmful effects of both smoking and drinking. I suppose the enforced regular, deep breathing which goes along with running inhibits the development of emphysema, one of the worst of the diseases promoted by smoking. I doubt that running has any inhibiting effect on cancer and probably not on the effect of nicotine on the heart, although a strong heart may be better able to take the shock of nicotine.

At any rate, I can gauge rather accurately how much I have smoked and how much I have had to drink the night before whenever I run. The smoking cuts down on my wind, although it seems to have that effect only for the first two or three miles.

The liquor, on the other hand, I feel in my legs. After a long night and numerous drinks, my legs feel dead when I begin to run and get worse as I go along, until the last mile or two of a fairly long run, they ache.

Someday, just possibly, I may quit smoking, since it is a habit with a very small feedback of pleasure and a very large feedback of guilt and possibility of damage to the body.

I don't think I'll quit drinking, however. It feels too good and it doesn't cost much.

Chapter Fourteen /

In spite of the smoking and drinking, the running continued to grow easier, both mentally and physically. The training effect which Dr. Cooper explains in his book seems to be a cumulative one; the better condition you attain, the easier it is to get in even better shape.

It was much easier to progress from jogging three miles a day to six to ten miles a day than it had been to go from scratch to three; the only problem, as the months went by, was to find enough time to get in all the running I wanted to do. It takes, for a slow, middle-aged runner with a scarred heart, about an hour and a half to run ten miles. Add to that another hour or so getting to the Y, dressing, showering, and dressing again and a heavy running schedule can account for nearly three hours out of the day.

However, by the time I had reached these distances early in 1970, I had decided that I would try to run in the Boston Marathon, an event which at that time was open to anyone with a deep and abiding desire to run twenty-six miles, 385 yards, no matter at what speed. The idea grew upon me gradually, nurtured I suppose by Andy Crichton and a couple of the other editors on *Sports Illustrated* who run in the marathon each year—and finish fairly well.

"It's difficult," Andy said. "But not impossible. You'll have to get in a lot of outdoor work and some on hills, but I think you may be able to do it. At least give it a try."

Jerry considered the idea of my running in a marathon ridiculous, but I thought that if I went at it slowly enough, I might be able to finish. Runners a good deal older than I have run in the marathon and finished well.

As I ran during that time, I did mental arithmetic, trying to decide what time I could project for myself if I did run at Boston. Running a distance on a small track like the one at the West Side Y means that you have to have something to think about, once you have reached the point where you are not primarily concerned simply with survival. During the first year, I spent all my time monitoring my own physical condition—how my heart felt, whether or not I would be able to keep up pace and breathe deeply enough to keep going, the ache in my knee or my ankle or the general deadness of my legs, and the feel of my feet in the running shoes.

But by the second year, except for rare occasions when I had a twinge of gout, I ran effortlessly and thought about a number of things, including stories I intended to write, other runners on the track going a better pace than mine, and the marathon.

I suppose I fell into the syndrome which can easily take over the neophyte jogger, no matter what his age or state of health. In the first few months, when I was trying only to defeat myself in the sense that I had to fight an overwhelming desire to quit jogging and start walking, I didn't pay much attention to the other runners on the various tracks where I tortured myself.

But as I got over the first pains of running, I became aware of the mini track meet going on around me every time I ran with other people on the track. I suppose the spirit of competition never dies and certainly in the men who had enough spirit, in their fifties and sixties, to run every day, the spirit was strong.

I stayed clear of it for a long time, actually. If a younger or better runner lapped me a few times during the course of my three miles, it never occurred to me to resent it. There were, of course, joggers who went along at about the same slow waddle that I used at first but I didn't even resent it when one of them, puffing and flailing his arms, finished his run in a blaze of glory by out-sprinting me in his last two laps. I wasn't interested in sprinting to the finish line; I was perfectly satisfied to reach it.

But as time passed I found myself changing. Runners who had lapped me when I started were going only a trifle faster and, as my heart and lungs quit laboring and engaging all the attention of my mind, I became more and more aware of them. And, of course, the stopwatch which I wore on a lanyard around my neck began to assume more and more importance.

The first runner I managed to pass was Bob Cooper, the attorney who runs despite the pain of a circulation blockage in his legs. I'm sure Bob was never aware that I was competing with him.

Much later, when I could do mental arithmetic as I ran, I worked out that Bob, and the little trail of runners who used him as a pacemaker, was running eleven-minute miles. Among the regulars who dropped in behind him for varying distances was a rather plump, balding man who ran in a gray sweat suit which looked for all the world like a set of old-fashioned long handles; a small, white-haired man with a quick, busy step; and a tall, thin man in his forties who seemed to have difficulty cutting his stride to match Bob's short, economical steps.

It took me over six months to reach the point where I could keep Bob's pace, but I never dropped in at the rear of his group, for some reason or other. I suppose it was because my pace never exactly matched his and at the time I was slowly increasing it, almost day by day. I remember that one day, when Bob and his followers came by me, I decided that I would see if I could pass them and did. After that I lapped him at long intervals, which grew shorter and shorter as I grew stronger.

I wasn't consciously competing then; it would have been a totally unfair race, even had Bob been aware of it. He was running from nine miles a day on up and I was running two or three. Later, when I was running as far as Bob, I felt much the same as he must have felt if he ever thought about it. When a jogger came on the track and took off at a pace a minute a mile faster than mine, I'd decide in my mind how far he was going.

"Two miles," I'd say to myself, then count his laps, adding one every time he passed me, subtracting one if I passed him. When he finished what I had come to feel was practically a sprint, I felt a warm sense of self-approbation, simply because I was on my way to six or seven or more miles.

Sometimes I would be counting laps for three or four other runners at the same time, keeping track of my own on the tallier I carried in my left hand, pushing in the plunger each time I passed the clock at one end of the track. It gave me something to do on the long runs and a way to avoid keeping track of laps in my mind—or being aware of how many more laps I had to run to finish the mileage I had set for myself.

I would make myself a promise not to look at the lap counter until after Runner X, who was passing me about every eighth lap, had finished and I knew how far he had gone. Then Runner Y would come on the track, going even faster than Runner X, and I would begin to count his laps; if a Runner Z came along, lapping me, too, I checked him.

With all the mental arithmetic going on in my mind, I could lose track of how far I had run; since the actual number of laps per mile at the West Side Y is 23.6, if I were going ten miles, I had to run 236 laps. On a good day, with a series of runners to keep track of other than myself, I have run 150 laps without looking at my lap counter. It makes the time pass.

Then, as time passed and I grew more aware of the competitive aspect of jogging, I began developing personal feuds with some of the other regulars on the track. I don't know if any of them were ever aware of me dogging their footsteps; I have a hunch they were, since I think all joggers react in the same way.

As I began consciously to compete, I would pick out

a runner a bit faster than I and set a time goal—so many weeks or months—to match his pace. At first, at the end of a run, I would decide to stay with him for the last half mile of my run, building in a strong finish, and try to pass him in the last two or three laps.

Sometimes he would accelerate when I did and make it impossible for me to pass him. Now and then, I would pass a runner and have him pass me back, looking ahead, paying no attention to me, but aware that he was passing me back.

I caught and passed a small, dark man I referred to mentally as the bank clerk and another, faster runner who was very tall with a tremendous stride, and set sail after a muscular, compact man who lost about fifteen pounds in the six months it took me to reach his speed and go beyond it. He had a square, tough face so that I always thought of him as a policeman, although I never found out either his name or his occupation.

Actually, I recognized most of the regulars from their shoes and the shape of their back and the rhythm of their stride; on a small track, whether you are passing or being passed, what you see is the rear of the other runners. It was only when I had finished running and was walking around the track to warm down that I looked at the faces of the other joggers.

There were, of course, many joggers I never caught and many I could not have caught had I been running in my prime, with a whole heart. I had enough sense to realize that the six-minute-mile men were far beyond my capabilities. Crichton, on the rare occasions when he ran indoors, ran on the outside of the track, flying along far faster than I can ever hope to and competing much more fiercely than I ever did.

While I labored slowly to dispose of the competition within the range of my physical strength, Andy took it as a personal insult if *anyone* passed him.

I used to admire Andy from a considerable distance, paddling along on the rail while he ran on the outside edge of the narrow track, whipping by the slower runners with an occasional exclamation of "Track!" when a slower runner happened to drift wide into his path. Now and again, he accelerated; if the West Side Y did not have banked turns, Andy, on a good day, might have gone out the window into Central Park from centrifugal force.

The competition, of course, is not good for a man in his fifties with a damaged heart, but it is a very seductive thing and something I still have to fight. Bob Cooper brought me back to my senses after I had reached the point where I was matching his mileage and after I had met him and most of his trailers.

I was running nine miles that day, passing Bob and his group rather often, when I suddenly became aware that I had someone on my tail. By then, this happened fairly often; after you have spent a long time on the same track, there are runners who discover that your speed is good for them for whatever distance they are going, so they fall in and go with you for a mile or two or more, but on that day, I hadn't picked up any trailers.

I was on the last two miles and I was going what, for me, seemed a rather brisk pace, probably something in the vicinity of eight minutes a mile. I felt good and strong and I began going faster and faster, but the runner behind me held on easily, even when I sprinted—

sprinted, for me—the last quarter of a mile.

I went by the finish line and punched my stopwatch and slowed to a stop and turned to see who had been going with me and it was Bob, not blowing at all.

"Nice pace, Tex," he said. "It's wonderful that you can do that for nine miles."

"I can't," I said. "I was just finishing."

"It's still remarkable," he said.

"Thanks," I told him. "I was a little surprised you finished so fast." (Fast. It's all a matter of comparison.)

"Once in a while I do that just to see how much I have left," Bob said. "I felt good today and my legs didn't bother me."

If his legs were all right, Bob could probably run me into the ground at any distance, any time he wanted to, but he is a gentle and thoughtful man. Crichton, who is not a notably modest man, told me later that before his legs began to slow him down, Bob would run step for step with him for as far as he wanted to go.

"You don't really have to run fast," Bob said that afternoon. "I think it's great that you do, but long, slow distance is just as good."

"I want to run in the Boston Marathon," I said, and was surprised at myself when I said it. I had been thinking about the marathon when I wasn't thinking about overtaking the next fastest runner at the Y, but I had never said to anyone that I was thinking about it.

"You don't mean that," Bob said.

"Yes, I do," I told him. "I just want to see how far I can go."

"Good luck," Bob said and grinned. "I hope you make it."

This was sometime in January 1970, after I had finished about sixteen months of jogging; you don't get ready to run a marathon starting in your fifties after a heart attack in eighteen months and the Boston Marathon takes place on Patriot's Day, which is a little after the middle of April.

I didn't know that; after I ran the twelve miles to celebrate the fourth anniversary of my heart attack, I honestly thought that the marathon would not be that tough.

The mental arithmetic I began doing then was not concerned with whether or not I would be able to run the twenty-six miles plus; I was trying to work out, at the pace I was running, whether I could finish under four hours.

I was running nine-minute miles consistently then, over distances up to ten miles, and finishing in no distress, except that my legs tired in the last mile or two, when I stepped up the pace.

Nine-minute miles, I thought, chugging along. Nine times twenty-six is 234 minutes. Four times sixty minutes is 240 minutes, so I would do twenty-six miles in six minutes under four hours, which leaves me six minutes to run 385 yards, and most of that downhill. I think I can do it.

By early April, I had convinced myself that, first, I could run twenty-six miles and, second, that I could run it fast enough not to disgrace myself completely.

What I had not taken into consideration, of course, is that, while the last quarter of a mile or so of the Boston Marathon is, indeed, downhill, a great deal of the other twenty-six miles, 385 yards, is uphill.

I was given an assignment in London on April 1, so I did not have a chance to test my ability to finish the marathon. On the day the marathon was run in Boston, I ran half the marathon distance in London, on the track at the Duke of York Headquarters.

I had intended to run at least twenty miles, but that day in London came on very cold and wet. I started running in the rain, ran through snow and sleet and finished up in cold sunshine, with blue hands, numb feet, and an overpowering desire to get back to my flat and a hot bath.

But I wasn't discouraged. I decided, after I had thawed out, that it had all worked out for the best. Another year would give me time to build up my stamina and cut down my time, so that I could run a respectable marathon.

Chapter Fifteen /

So early in 1970 I began serious training for the marathon, but told no one. I stretched out the distances and increased the pace and felt very good, especially knowing that it would be another year before I had to run in Boston.

I ran outdoors whenever I could. Once, in Los Angeles, I ran outdoors at a YMCA that did not have an indoor track. What they had was a map of the neighborhood, giving you directions on where to go if you wanted to run one, two, three or more miles.

"Run south on Sepulveda to Washington Street," the directions said, for four miles. "Turn right on Washington to Culver and right on Culver to Adams. Turn right on Adams and run back to the Y."

So I set off in my running gear one morning, running along Sepulveda toward the airport, which wasn't far away. I felt a little embarrassed, but since the Y running routes were mimeographed, I figured that the people in the neighborhood must be used to seeing joggers trundling by.

Two young girls greeted me as I went along. They were passing me slowly and they said, "Good morning," and I nodded. They watched me curiously for a few moments as they went by and I smiled to show that I could have been running much faster if I had wanted to.

"The church is on the next corner on the right," one of them said, rather mysteriously. I felt I had to say something to that.

"Aaargh," I said, noncommittally.

I ran along the beach at Miami Beach, inadvertently running much farther than I had intended. I had found a long stretch of waterfront with a walk behind it and I asked the lifeguard on duty on the beach how far it was to a distant pier.

"About a mile," he said. "And no hills."

"Thank you," I said, a bit sourly. I wasn't that afraid of hills.

I ran back and forth to the pier three times, which I calculated at six miles and it took me about twenty minutes longer than I thought it should and left me a good deal more exhausted.

As I walked by the lifeguard on my way back to my car, he stopped me.

"Hey," he said, "I made a mistake. It's a mile to the pier the other way. That one's a mile and a half."

"And no hills," I told him. "Thanks."

I ran in parking lots, on city streets, in place in hotel and motel rooms all over the United States. I ran around practice fields in most of the training camps of the National Football League, much to the amusement of the players.

Once, in New Orleans doing a story on the Saints, I ran at their training camp, laboring along through thick grass and avoiding a pit bulldog belonging to Doug Atkins, the thirty-nine-year-old defensive end for the Saints. Doug had tied the dog to the fence surrounding the training area and each time I went by him I gave him a wide berth, although he showed no real interest in me.

Each time I went by, Doug shook his head at me dolefully.

"It's too *late*, Tex," he said. "Man, don't you know it's too late?"

"Not for me," I puffed and went on.

Later, in the dressing room, he introduced me to Rebel, the pit bull, so that Rebel would look on me as a friend when I ran the next day. Rebel looked at me dolefully, then got up and made his way painfully to a cool corner and lay down again. I was sweating profusely, but I hadn't thought it was that bad.

"What's the matter with Rebel?" I asked Doug.

"I matched him with a big ol' police dog last night," Doug said. "Reb woulda killed him if he had any teeth. As it was, after the big ol' police dog chewed him up a little, he got the police dog down and was gummin' him pretty bad when we stopped it."

"You mean Rebel doesn't have any teeth?"

"Nope," Doug said. "He lost 'em a couple years ago."

Atkins matched Rebel with other dogs whenever he

could find an owner willing to pit his dog, which was reasonably often. I looked at Rebel with more respect but a good deal less fear.

Dogs, of course, are one of the hazards of running outdoors, for two reasons. Most dogs react to the sight of a full-grown man trotting along the road with about the same emotion as if the man were a full-grown cat. And as often as not, if the dog's owner is along, the owner reacts with anger toward the runner, not the dog.

One morning, running in Golden Gate Park in San Francisco, I was set upon by a small black French poodle. French poodles, as a group, are usually good-natured dogs with a sophisticated outlook on the frailties of man, but this one was an exception to the rule, unfortunately.

He barked for a while, running along beside me and yapping enthusiastically, but offering no violence. He was not a very big dog, but even small dogs, I have learned rather painfully, can bring blood when they bite.

I paid no attention to him, slogging along steadily and trying to enjoy the pleasant scenery, hoping he would grow tired and go away, but he drew courage from my ignoring him and finally began making little forays at my heels, snarling and snapping.

I took that for a little while, then turned and yelled, "Bug off!" which may not be the proper thing to say at such a time, but it was all I could think of then.

It worked well enough, because the poodle yiped in terror and took off into the bushes.

I went on peacefully for another hundred yards, congratulating myself on having handled a difficult situation with aplomb and dispatch. Then I became aware of footsteps behind me. I thought at first that it was another jogger going a bit faster than I, but I found out otherwise quickly enough.

"Stop, you son of a bitch!" a female voice howled from about two points off my starboard beam and I looked around.

A rather elderly, thin woman was running along after me, carrying the dog in her arms, with her hair beginning to straggle around her face.

"You mean me, ma'am?" I said, speeding up a bit.

"You see anyone else around?"

I looked around, still stepping up the pace, and she was right. I was the only person she could have been talking to.

"No, ma'am," I said and lengthened my stride a bit more. By now I was going at what, for me, was a pretty fair clip and what, for an elderly lady carrying a small dog, should have been nearly impossible.

"Why did you yell at Pierre?" she said, gaining ground so that she was just about even with me.

"Pierre?"

She shook the damned poodle, which appeared to be more tired than his mistress.

"Him," she said. "He wasn't hurting you."

"No," I replied, slowing down a bit so that I would be able to finish my six miles. "But he was about to."

"How do you know?"

"How do you know he wasn't?"

"Pierre has never bitten a runner in his life," she said indignantly. I was a little surprised to note that she wasn't even breathing hard. She had a nice, easy stride, even encumbered by having to carry Pierre.

"Has he had many opportunities?" I asked.

She ran along beside me for another fifty yards thinking about that and I slowed down a little more, not for the sake of companionship, but to save myself for a good hard closing mile.

"Three or four," she said. "He likes to bark at them, but I don't think he ever bit one."

"Maybe he doesn't like me," I said.

"I'll put him down," she said. "Let's see what he does."

She seemed to have gotten over her spell of ill temper, but Pierre, bouncing up and down in her arms, didn't look any friendlier.

"Why don't you just stop and let me get a couple of hundred yards ahead before you put him down?" I asked, but she shook her head.

"No," she replied. "I think it's important to find out if he *will* bite. I mean, if he does, then I'll have to think of some way to cure him of it."

"You don't mind if I would prefer not to be the guinea pig?"

"I think you owe it to Pierre," she said. "You were the one who scared him."

"Or vice versa," I said.

"Pooh," she said, running easily and well and obviously able to keep on. "How could a little dog like this scare a man as big as you are?"

"I'm cowardly," I said. I looked at her to see if she was showing signs of flagging, but she was still breathing as easily as I, or maybe easier. I had gone about four miles by then; she had gone maybe a quarter of a mile, but she looked good for a lot more.

"Are you a runner?" I asked her.

"Not really," she said. "A couple of miles a morning."

"You look good," I said. "Nice stride."

"Thanks," she said. "How far you going?"

"Six," I told her. "You and Pierre willing."

"I'll put him down," she said and did. He trotted along with us a few seconds, then went off on his own. Most dogs are unable to run the distance a man can; if you have a pet and expect him to run with you over any real distance, you may kill him. For that matter, a man can run a horse to death, too.

She ran along with me for another half mile, during the course of which she said that Pierre always ran a few steps with her, then went off on his own.

"How about the three or four other runners he barked at?"

"They just ran on," she said. "I guess they knew he was harmless."

"I suppose you're right," I said. "I just thought he was getting too close." We had turned around and were jogging back the way we had come and Pierre came out of the bushes and bit me on the ankle. It wasn't a severe bite and left only a scratch and I liked his mistress well enough by then not to kick Pierre into orbit, but I was a bit irritated.

"Well," she said, after I had used a few words not ordinarily used in the presence of elderly ladies, "at least we know."

"Know what?"

"He bites people he doesn't like," she said. "I'm sorry."

Well, it didn't hurt that much, really. I ran in Golden Gate Park several times after that, but I never ran into Pierre or his mistress, thank goodness.

In Central Park, the dogs are much more tolerant than Pierre. For one thing, I suppose they are accustomed to being among people all the time and for another, most of them are on leash. But they are difficult in another way.

While I am not a dog hater (once, many years ago in another state and another time, I raised Scottish terriers), I think they definitely have their place and Manhattan is not it.

No dog can get enough exercise in Manhattan to be really healthy, to begin with. Secondly, I have never considered dog excrement any more pleasant than the human variety and when you are running in the roads in Central Park, you become very much aware of how many non-constipated dogs inhabit this crowded borough. If the Manhattan dogs, as a rule, don't bite it is probably because they are far too busy defecating in the street.

If you walk regularly in Manhattan, you instinctively look where you walk. When you're jogging or running, your reactions have to be much quicker and it is easier to get distracted and not look at all.

Once around Central Park is a little less than seven miles and I doubt that there is a stretch of a hundred yards in which no dog has left its mark. Of course, the same thing is true of Manhattan's city streets; they are foul from the Bronx to the Battery.

However, the peril of running in Central Park is not primarily that of stepping in dog leavings and earning a bit of unwanted luck. Nor is there any danger of a runner being mugged, since even the most moronic mugger has enough sense to know that a jogger, wearing shorts, a singlet, running shoes, and a pained expression, has no place to conceal any valuables. Maybe a mugger might covet my stopwatch, swinging from my neck, but it would be much simpler to mug an old man walking along than to run me down to take my stopwatch.

The kids are the major hazard in Central Park. Little ones who toddle into your path and subteeners who feel that almost nothing in their repulsive lives can match the comedy of watching a middle-aged man in shorts running.

If a dog harasses you, you can yell at it and kick it, but society frowns on full-grown men who quit jogging long enough to boot a sassy brat in the butt.

"Hey, looka da ol geezer," one once yelled to his repulsive friends as I was running along, minding my own business. "Get a load a dat!"

This small group of hellions had been happily engaged in playing among themselves or dismembering insects when I trotted by them; they considered me better entertainment. They followed me for two or three blocks, howling insults or running in front of me making faces and noise. I made a few ineffectual swipes at the boldest when they came near me, but luckily I never hit one. I would probably have been sued if I had.

The younger generation, to my everlasting gratitude, is as short on condition as it is on manners, so that when a runner is beset by small beasts like these, it is only for a block or two. They run out of breath about as quickly as they run out of imagination, which is quickly.

Most of the joggers, or runners, who use Central Park as a training ground, dress at the West Side Y, which is just across Central Park West from the park. So you run into quite a few serious runners there, most of them much faster than the joggers, who stay inside on the small track.

So the competition is tougher and it is over longer distances.

It was well along in my second year before I could run fast enough to even try to compete. I mean, for a long time, I was content to run on the bicycle path, which is a little over a mile and a half around and which is inhabited by irate bicyclers and slow runners.

The guys on the bikes seem to think they own the bicycle path, for some reason. They never give a jogger the right of way; occasionally they become insulting, like the old gaffer who yelled to me to get the unmentionable out of the way when there were only the two of us on the bicycle path and he had all the room in the world to avoid me.

I thought seriously of bumping him as he went by, but I suppose that would have been too drastic a riposte to a mild insult. So I just called him a few choice names and watched his neck turn red as he pedaled away.

When I started running on the long circuit around the park, aside from children, runners were the most obnoxious. There was one in particular who irked me.

You dress in the West Side Y on small stools in front of your locker and when it is crowded the stools are hard to come by. When you get a stool, you mark it as yours by putting the wire basket with your running gear on it; then, if you have to leave to go to the john or attend to some other necessary function, you can expect to have the stool and the locker waiting for you on your return.

Several times, I had marked my locker and my seat

with my basket and returned to find my basket on the floor and this objectionable red-haired type sitting on the stool. These incidents occurred at long-drawn-out intervals and I never caught him in the act of putting my basket on the floor, so I could hardly take issue with him.

I knew he was a runner by his gear, but I never saw him on the small indoor track; it was not until I began running outdoors and until I moved up from the bicycle path to the grand circuit that I saw him.

He was, I must admit, a good runner. He was tall and lean and his red hair was flecked plentifully with gray, but he ran with the easy lope of the practiced long-distance runner and for a long time I considered him out of my class, which indeed he was.

Then I missed him for a month or so and asked Cooper, who knows every runner at the Y, where he was.

"Sick," Cooper said. "I think he had pneumonia, or something like that."

"I hope he's all right," I said, hypocritically. I didn't wish him any real illness, just something that would slow him down.

I saw him again a couple of weeks later. I suppose he had been running wherever he lived, coming back slowly, but I had not seen him in the park and I saw him first sitting serenely on the stool where my basket had been a few moments ago. I was sure by now that he was the one who appropriated my stool, but I figured that I could put up with it from a sick man.

Then I ran into him as I began my six-and-a-half-mile jog; he passed me about a half a mile out, as I was running along Central Park South , heading for the turn up Fifth Avenue.

He went by running stylishly, and nodded to me as he passed, smiling with a disgusting air of superiority, as if he were one of the titled heads of the running game and I was a peasant.

I speeded up for a few moments to stay close to him, then decided that it would be foolish to try to run with him. I knew he was much faster.

I went on my way, avoiding the occasional urchin and the not-so-occasional dog sign, not expecting to see the red-haired man again until I returned to the locker room. I was wrong.

I saw him ahead of me when I made the turn on to Central Park West, the home stretch back to the Y. He was a couple of hundred yards ahead of me, but he had slowed a good deal and, to my surprise, I found I was overtaking him. I put on a small burst of what passes for speed with me as I went by and smiled smugly and nodded at him.

Two hundred yards farther on, he passed me; for the last mile, we took turns passing each other and we finished almost in a dead heat, sprinting away grimly. It would be hard to say who won, since we finished at different spots; I thought I had won when he slowed down after passing *his* finishing post and I'm sure he figured he had won, since he was ahead by a couple of strides at the time.

In the locker room later, he nodded to me and said, "Nice run."

He swiped stools from someone else after that, and after he got fit again, I never passed him. At the time, I was not trying to beat individual competitors. My principal rival was the stopwatch and I made up ground on that slowly, but surely.

Chapter Sixteen /

In December of 1970, by the time the regular season of the National Football League drew to a close, I was in better shape than I had ever been in my life, running from six to ten miles, five days a week, and running faster.

I had been trying, with fair success, to cut down on smoking, keeping a record of how many cigarettes I smoked each day. On good days, I would smoke only five or six; under writing pressure, it would go up to a pack or so, but I was still running well and I felt more and more confident that I would be able to finish the twenty-six-mile-plus marathon route, maybe in under four hours.

Crichton goes on the wagon for three months before

every marathon and I decided I would do that, too. But first, with playoffs, conference championship games, and the Super Bowl coming up, I decided to take a couple of weeks off, which was a mistake.

I missed two weeks running and spent the two weeks drinking too much and smoking too much and gaining weight. By the time I got back to a fairly regular regime, I had gained about eight pounds and it was difficult to run five miles, but I thought that I still had time to get fit before the marathon, which was scheduled for April 19, 1971.

After you have established a discipline of running, it is much easier to regain a good level of fitness than it is to reach the same level from scratch. Within a month, I was back up to ten miles, then I missed a week with the gout and another week on an assignment in San Antonio, Texas, where I was raised and where I have far too many convivial drinking companions.

Still, I felt strong and although time was growing short, I was not far out of peak condition. I had cut down on smoking and cut down on drinking and was near my best running weight, when I was slowed down again by an assignment. By now, I was beginning to doubt that I would be able to run the whole twenty-six miles; you can't prepare for a marathon in the short time then left to me.

Besides, the sponsors of the marathon threw me—and all the slow joggers like me—a curve by making it a rule that you had to have run a marathon in under four hours before you would be eligible as an official entry in Boston. Surprisingly, several of the really fine marathon runners who would be competing with a hope of winning objected seriously to this restriction.

One of the charms of the Boston race is its air of informality; it is a serious, tough competition, but most of the competitors and their friends enjoy it as a pleasant outing where old friends turn up and old stories are rehashed ad infinitum.

For a while, some of the top competitors threatened to take off their numbers—numbers issued as evidence of an official entry—and run without identification, but eventually that scheme died a natural death.

"Don't worry about it," Crichton told me. "Every year there are a lot of guys who show up and run without numbers. They aren't supposed to, but with over a thousand runners up there, no one ever stops them."

This was in February and around the first of the month I had gotten a note from Dr. Ted Kirkham, the head of the medical staff for Time-Life, Inc. He asked me if I would participate in a study to be conducted by the Division of Human Ecology at Cornell University Medical College under the sponsorship of the National Heart and Lung Institute.

I talked to him about the project and found that it was to be an in-depth investigation of coronary heart disease, using 150 volunteers from the New York area, and designed to find out, if possible, the predisposing factors leading to a heart attack.

"You will have to spend a night, a day, and a night at the hospital," Dr. Kirkham told me. "For twenty-four hours, you'll carry a tape recorder attached to leads which will in effect give the study group a twenty-four-hour electrocardiogram under varying conditions. After that, about once every six months, you'll be asked to carry another tape recorder in the form of a brief case for a twenty-four-hour EKG under the average conditions of a day of work."

"How about running?" I asked him.

"Sure," he said. "If it's a small track, the recorder will pick up the signal easily enough."

I agreed to take part and forgot about the whole thing until three weeks later.

A series of assignments out of the city made training difficult, so that I was not running well and I knew that I would have to work hard during March and April if I hoped to make even a remotely respectable attempt in the marathon.

I had not run in over a week when I got a brief note informing me that I would be expected to turn up at the Cornell Medical Center, which is only a few blocks from my apartment in Manhattan, by seven in the evening on the following Tuesday, some five days later.

When I showed up, with my overnight bag, I was assigned a room in a suite with a pleasant man who had worked for the telephone company for a long time. An intern came into the room after we had been there for a half hour and told us that we would be awakened at seven the next morning and left a thick sheaf of questionnaires to be filled out.

I decided I would go out for a cup of coffee before settling down with the questionnaires and I managed to slip and fall on the steps leading out of the building. When I got up, I felt a sharp pain in my left forefinger and looked at it to find that I had dislocated the finger at the second joint so that it made an L as I looked at it. I pulled it sharply and it snapped back into place and I had my coffee. The finger did not hurt much then.

I went back up to the suite and worked on the questionnaires for two hours; they covered my medical history from birth, my work, my outlook on life, and just about everything else that could conceivably be of any interest to a doctor. They were, in fact, an indication of how thorough the examination for this study would be and I doubt seriously that any study will be based on more complete data.

When I had finished filling out the forms, I went into the bedroom of the suite and found my roommate was already asleep. He had arrived before I had and finished his homework early; I knew he was asleep because he was snoring.

I don't mind snoring; I spent five years in the merchant marine and a good deal of time, one way or another, sleeping in athletic dormitories where snorers are endemic. But this gentle, considerate man, in what I suppose were his early sixties, had made snoring one of the great arts.

He had great range and feeling and good volume and a truly remarkable talent for improvisation. If you could play the snore in a Dixieland band, he would have made Louis Armstrong look like a novice. Most snorers are fairly regular in their production so that you can expect a snore at intervals of X seconds and grow accustomed to the rhythm. My friend had no rhythm and finally I retired to the living room of the suite and slept on the couch.

Promptly at seven, an intern knocked on the door. Both of us were awake and the intern, carrying a heavy load of electronic equipment, wired my roommate first, and then me.

To do this, he first shaved the hair off my chest, then attached leads in four different spots, so that my heart was being monitored by a small, square box which I carried on my hip, suspended from my shoulder by a strap.

For the next twenty-four hours, the little black box would record every reaction my heart would have to the various tests conducted. It was not hard to grow used to; after about twenty-two hours I hardly knew it was there.

After both of us had been attached and checked out, we went out with our intern for the first confrontation of the day. When we reached the office of the doctor who conducted the first tests, we found two other volunteers there.

One of them was from Time-Life, Inc., but he was from the advertising segment of the operation and I did not know him. We sat and listened while the doctor explained to us what the study hoped to accomplish.

It is a good idea and I hope that it arrives at some worthwhile conclusions. The 150 men—all volunteers—involved in the study are separated into three groups.

All of them are executives in New York, subject, supposedly, to about the same amount of pressure in their professional and social lives. Fifty are men who, by the medical records kept by their companies, are, by presently known criteria, unlikely to suffer a heart attack. All of the subjects come from big corporations that keep complete enough records so that the doctors involved in the survey would have enough data to make an informed guess as to the future of the subject as far as heart and lung disease are concerned.

Fifty more of the 150 are men who may or may not have a heart attack, and the other fifty—including, obviously, me—are men who are likely to have heart attacks.

By keeping a continuous electrocardiogram for twenty-four hours under varying conditions, there is a possibility that the doctors in charge of the survey will be able to find a pattern which may help other doctors in the future predict heart trouble before it gives any sign at present decipherable.

If the rest of the 150 are comparable to me and the other three men who were with me, they are a fairly representative cross section of middle-aged, reasonably successful people. None of us were extraordinary. I suppose I was the most athletic, at the stage in life when we were picked, but I was not the most successful nor the most stress-ridden.

After the idea of the survey had been explained, we began a series of exhaustive tests. We had our blood pressure taken over and over again, enough blood drawn to start a blood bank. We were tested lying down, standing up, walking, sitting, and on a treadmill, walking at 1.7 miles an hour for two minutes up a 12 percent grade.

We didn't get anything to eat for a long time, then we had lunch in the hospital cafeteria and I ate more than I really wanted, simply to cheer up the nurse who was with us by then. The food was not very good, but I knew that she had to eat it every day, so I put away a large portion of whatever it was with as much enthusiasm as I could muster.

Late in the afternoon, we walked to another of what by now seemed to be an unending number of small rooms with testing personnel waiting, for a truly comprehensive physical. This was the kind of physical you get each year, if you work for Time-Life, Inc. or any other really big corporation, and it includes blood tests, urinalyses, blood pressure, EKG, and all the other usual procedures.

By this time, the four of us were fairly well-acquainted. We sat in a small anteroom, waiting for our turns in the examining room, and worked crossword puzzles, thoughtfully provided by the people in charge.

When I went into the examining room, I was a bit surprised to find that the doctor who would examine me was a woman. She was in her early thirties, attractive, and very businesslike.

We went through the usual procedure. She hit me on the knee with a rubber hammer and I kicked out, and she peered into my ears and down my throat and listened to my heart and lungs saying, "Take a deep breath. Another, another, another."

She felt for my liver and found it and I began to grow a bit uneasy. I am not an overly modest man, but I have been through many company physicals and I know the procedure as well as most doctors.

So I was not surprised when she said, "Stand up. Drop your shorts and bend over."

After you have spent some eight hours being tapped, listened to, punctured, and palpated by a wide assortment of nurses and interns, you tend to become a bit depersonalized, so that you move more or less like an automaton through whatever trials are offered. The ambience of the hospital tends to take away your independence; the atmosphere of complete dependence upon the powers that be is an easy one to become used to. Most people are happy in an environment where they can do what they are told without the necessity of making a conscious choice or assuming a conscious responsibility.

I suppose that if I had had to undergo this particular indignity in the first series of tests I took that day, I might have objected, although there is no rational reason why I should have. The doctor-patient relationship in this situation is about as impersonal as it can get. At any rate, I did not question this female doctor's right to investigate the possibility of my prostate being something less than up to par.

So I dropped my shorts and bent over, when she told me to.

"You must feel a good deal like Myra Breckinridge," I said, as she pulled on her rubber gloves.

"Not really," she said. "Actually, you're lucky, you know."

"How is that?"

"I have very small hands," she said.

After she had finished with me, I went back to the small waiting room, and in a little while she came out and talked to us about what had happened during the day and what the background of the survey included.

It was interesting and informative and she obviously knew a great deal about the history of research into coronary heart disease and what might lie in the future. She gave all of us cards to carry in our wallets, saying that we were participating in the study and that the doctors listed on the card should be contacted should any of us become ill.

She was reassuring, though.

"If there was anything seriously wrong with any of you, we would probably know it by now," she said. "So far as I know, nothing is. Of course, we'll send a full report to your respective doctors when we get the results of all the tests and have had time to evaluate them, which should be in about two or three weeks. Then, in about six months, or maybe a little longer, we'll ask you to spend a day with a transistorized piece of equipment which will allow us to keep another twenty-four-hour electrocardiogram during a normal day's activity."

All of us, of course, were still wired to our recording machines, as we had been all day. After the briefing, we left in a group, shepherded by the two interns who had been with us intermittently all day, headed for a restaurant, where we were to have dinner on the research foundation.

The restaurant was chosen not by any gourmet standard but by the fact that it was almost exactly a mile from where we had had our final physical and the little box we carried on our hips was interested in how our hearts would react to a walk of a mile. I never found out specifically how mine held up under the strain, but at the pace we walked I certainly felt no discomfort.

Unfortunately, the restaurant was a family-style Hungarian restaurant. We created a minor flurry of interest as we waited for our table. The four patients, including me, looked a bit like a delegation from Mars or Venus, come to earth to sample Terran civilization. All of us had wires sprouting from our shirt fronts and entering the little black boxes on our hips and the other customers looked at us with the guarded curiosity with which most New Yorkers regard anything out of the ordinary.

When we were seated, the senior intern told us that dinner was on Dr. Lawrence E. Hinkle, Jr., who was in charge of the research.

"You can have two drinks," he said. "Then you can have anything you want to eat and as much as you like."

We had the two drinks, then took a vote to decide whether we should have two or three more, at our own expense. First we checked with the interns to find out if more than two drinks might, in some arcane way, destroy the validity of the whole program. They said no, so we had two more drinks each.

Then we ate an abominable dinner, which may have done more to irritate my heart than anything that had happened to me since I had had the coronary. The company, however, was pleasant and we had wine with dinner so that by the time we had finished I felt fairly mellow.

After dinner we went to a movie, a French movie with subtitles, which must have been reflected in my EKG as a two-hour nap. I had considerable difficulty keeping my eyes open.

We had the same effect on the people waiting to get into the movie as we had had on the patrons of the Hungarian restaurant. They looked at us with quiet suspicion, regarding the little black boxes as possible explosives, but too afraid to commit themselves to any kind of positive action to protest.

When the movie dragged to its inconclusive and uninteresting finish, we walked back the measured mile to our suites in the hospital and I retired to the living room, leaving my snoring friend in complete possession of the bedroom.

I did not sleep particularly well. There was a coffee table next to the bed, where I deposited the little black box. By now my chest was sore from the attachments feeding information into the box and whenever I wanted to turn over during the night I had to arrange all the wires so that they would neither strangle me nor pull the box off the table.

So for most of the night I read. I don't remember the book, but I do remember that by the time I turned off the light it was the early hours of the morning and I knew that I would again be awakened at the crack of dawn so that I could be disconnected from the box and set free.

One of the interns had put a new tape in the box in midafternoon, and had checked to make sure that everything was in working order before my roommate and I went to sleep.

After I had finally fallen into a fitful sleep, not exactly lulled by the snores of my friend in the next room, I woke up almost immediately when I turned over suddenly on the couch and disconnected one of the leads. I connected it again as best I could and debated whether I should get up and go to the john.

I did, at last, creating some new and, I hope, interesting patterns on my EKG, then slept for about two hours before one of the interns woke me and took off all my attachments.

"Thanks," he said, as I dressed. "We really enjoyed being with you."

"It was fun," I said. "Anyway, it was different."

Chapter Seventeen /

For the next three weeks, I averaged a little more than five miles a day on the track and regained much of the condition I had lost. I was running easily, not trying for speed, using the LSD principle of most joggers. LSD is not a drug; it means long, slow distance. It is, undoubtedly, the wisest way for anyone over thirty-five to train, since it puts much less strain on the heart than running at or near capacity.

I put in one ten-mile run and felt good at the finish, and by the middle of March, with the marathon seven weeks away, I felt reasonably sure that I would be able to go fifteen or twenty miles, barring unseasonably hot weather or a head wind.

Then, a few days before my fifty-sixth birthday, I got

a phone call from my doctor, Jerry. Unfortunately, he had called my wife at home before he called me.

Jerry had received the report from the heart-study tests and he suggested that I come in for an immediate checkup. I am still not quite sure why, since he certainly was not equipped to give me a more thorough testing than I had had at the Cornell Medical Research Center.

The report, to put it bluntly, was not good. It was a detailed, single-spaced letter a little over four pages long, giving the results of all of the tests I had taken, most of them good enough, but the next to last paragraph and the one before that were not exactly designed to encourage me to run in the marathon, or, for that matter, to run far enough to catch a bus. I had, of course, detailed the amount of running I was doing on the preliminary reports I had filled in.

"In our opinion Mr. Maule has coronary heart disease, as manifested by the syndrome of a past myocardial infarction," the report said in summary. "He apparently was in cardiac failure during and after the infarction. At the present time his cardio-thoracic ratio on the chest x-ray is at the upper limits of normal, suggesting that he has some cardiac dilatation even though clinical evidence of congestive heart failure was not present at the time of our examination. He has continuing serious abnormalities of his standard electrocardiogram. His cardiac recordings indicate that he has multifocal VPCs (premature ventricular contractions) at a frequency of more than 10 per 1,000 complexes. They also indicate that these VPCs do not disappear during sleep or during physical activity.

"All of these findings, in our experience, carry with

them a high risk of the sudden development of a fatal dysrhythmia. While we do not think that Mr. Maule should necessarily interrupt his ordinary activities, we do believe that it is unwise for him to participate in strenuous exercise which might increase the risk that such a dysrhythmia would develop."

Since I had run five miles already on the morning I got that cheerful bit of news from Jerry, I was not immediately convinced that the diagnosis in the report was necessarily right. My wife, who hasn't run a total of five miles in the years we have been married, was sure that I had better slow down to a walk if I hoped to survive long enough to get home.

I went through another series of tests at Jerry's office, which revealed exactly what the research group had found out; I have premature ventricular contractions, which feel more like a skipped heart beat than an extra one, which is what they are. But I knew that my EKGs in my annual physicals at Time-Life, Inc. had shown extra beats for a long time.

After Jerry had convinced himself that the report of the premature beats was true, he warned me very seriously, with my wife listening tearfully, not to run any more. I listened to him doubtfully, but I agreed to hold off at least a week, while he checked the effect of a medication he gave me to help the gall bladder condition, which had kicked up a little.

"It's possible that that can trigger the premature contractions," he said. "Try this medication for a week and come back."

I did and the second examination showed fewer extra beats, but I was still running in an extra tick now and then and Jerry insisted that I should not run. I agreed to cut down on my mileage, but I told him that I was not going to quit entirely.

"After all," I told my wife later, "I have survived over five years since my heart attack and I feel good. My blood pressure is down and no matter what Jerry or the report says, I can still run over five miles without any discomfort. Hell, I couldn't do that *before* I had the heart attack. And I am not convinced that the doctors know anything about the effect of exercise on a heart like mine."

I had not run for a week by then, and I decided to start again, but I had to promise Dorothy that I would at least consult Dr. Kirkham, the Time-Life, Inc. doctor, before I did. Dr. Kirkham is a cardiologist and I called him and asked if he had read the report; he had. I told him how I felt about it and he asked me to wait a few more days before I began running, so that he could discuss the report with the doctors at Cornell Medical.

I saw him in his office two days later and we went over the report carefully.

Dr. Kirkham was much more reassuring than the report had been. I pointed out to him that I had had extra beats for a long time and had been running with no ill effects—quite the opposite—for over two years.

"I have survived quite a while on this program," I said. "And I feel a lot better than I did before I began running. I would like to keep on running."

"I talked it over at length with Dr. Hinkle," Dr. Kirkham said. "We really have no evidence of any kind on the effect the amount of running you do has on a post-cardiac patient, simply because I don't know any other post-cardiac patients who have taken that much exercise. So

I can't tell you with any degree of precision either to go on or to quit."

He smiled and shrugged his shoulders.

"I suppose what you are doing is exploring new medical frontiers," he said. "So I don't know anyone who can advise you one way or the other."

"But would you say the odds are as good one way as the other?"

"As far as we know," he said.

So I started running again. I cut back to three miles a day for several weeks and I was much, much more aware of my heartbeat than I had ever been before, but I still felt strong, despite the report and despite Jerry's advice. My wife was worried about the running for a while, but as I kept on with no noticeable ill effects, she gradually got over her concern.

The report did not worry me as much as it might a more apprehensive man; I am not by nature a worrier and I didn't worry in the weeks after I had read it. I thought about it for a long time after my interview with Dr. Kirkham, trying to weigh the pros and cons. I finally arrived at the conclusion that nothing had changed from the time before I had read the report and the time after except that I was aware that, according to one unsubstantiated opinion, running might kill me quickly.

However, if that were true, it seemed reasonable that, considering the amount of jogging I had done, I should have been long dead. So I ran and slowly built up the distance again.

The jogging was not as pleasant as it had been; running is difficult enough under the best of circumstances, but when it is complicated by your keeping a close watch on how your heart is reacting, it is rather unpleasant.

Early on, I had occasionally had slight pain in my chest when I jogged, but nothing serious enough to make me stop and nothing like the agonizing pain of angina pectoris. I had only once had a touch of angina, but I have read a good deal about it, and I'm sure I would recognize the pain if it should occur. Certainly, the pain I felt when I had the heart attack must have been very similar, since it came from the same cause, the diminution of the supply of blood to the heart.

When I had volunteered for the study group, I must confess that I had looked forward to getting a glowing report on the strength of my rebuilt heart. When the report seemed to say almost precisely the opposite, I was, for a week or so—and understandably—rather depressed.

But I got over that as I kept on jogging and felt the same sense of well-being that I had been feeling for over a year. I am not trying to say that the doctors don't know what they are talking about. Indeed, by the time you read this, they may well have been proved right and my running days—*all* my days—may be over.

But I didn't feel like that as I picked up my training routine again. After a few weeks, I quit listening to the rhythm of my heart and waiting for a pain in my chest to warn me to slow down. The pain didn't come and if my heart beat an extra beat now and then I didn't notice it, especially when I was finishing a six-mile run. When I tired, it was my legs that felt it, not my heart and lungs, and I knew why my legs tired. Too much vodka and tonic the night before.

Of course, I do not recommend the same procedure for

everyone. And I actually *did* take it easy, in that I was running good distances, but going slowly, staying well within my limit so that I never became exhausted. I cut my mile times down from an average of nine minutes to nine and a half and sometimes ten minutes per mile. You get the same training effect, nearly, at the slower pace, and your heart can jog along with you, instead of racing.

I didn't worry if someone passed me, or try to pass them back. After a week or two, I quit running with the stopwatch to avoid the temptation, when I felt good, to speed up at the end of a long run.

For a while I took my pulse frequently, waiting for the skip that marks an extra beat. The extra beat comes quickly at the end of a regular beat, so that there is a longer interval between that beat and the next, and I found them often enough.

I took my pulse after running, to try to find out if it was too fast; Dr. Cooper, and some others, have worked out a scale of exertion based upon the rate of the pulse, geared to age.

Most of them agree that the maximum pulse rate a man can attain during exercise comes down with age. For instance, a teen-ager can exercise violently enough and long enough for his heart to beat some 200 times plus per minute. In my age bracket, the maximum rate is around 160 beats per minute and in my age bracket, with a scarred heart, probably something less than that.

Actually, to gain a training effect—an effect which, over time, will improve the performance of the heart and lungs—I had to reach a much lower rate of 120 to 130 beats a minute.

For a couple of weeks, I would stop after a run and

check my heartbeat with a finger on the artery at the side of my neck, waiting rather anxiously to see if I had forced the beat too high, or if there were a large number of extra beats.

Oddly enough, after a long run I found no extra beats, despite what the Cornell report had said. Of course, during the course of that series of tests, I was never required to run or to take any more exercise than the two-minute stint on the treadmill and the one-mile walk from the movie. After a good run, the pulse in the side of my neck was strong and regular, never too fast. And the recovery rate was well within the limits recommended by the jogging books.

But it is not easy to shake off the kind of fear engendered by a report which says so plainly that your heart is faulty and you may die any moment by overtaxing it. There were a few nights when I found sleep not easily come by and lay quietly feeling each time my heart beat and each time it beat once too often. Counting heartbeats makes for a long and sleepless night, so I usually gave up an essentially fruitless pursuit and turned on my bedside light and read.

Familiarity at last breeds, not contempt, but resignation to a condition like mine. One day after a good run, I did not bother to check my pulse and within a few weeks I didn't think about it any more. My heart responded to exercise as easily as it had ever done and I began to think of other things during the course of a run.

One of the things I began to think about again was the marathon.

With all the interruptions in training I had had and with the major blow of the report, I knew that it would be impossible for me to run in it and finish, but I began to toy with the idea of running anyway.

Of course, after any kind of layoff, it is extremely important to work back into good condition slowly. Whenever I am forced to miss jogging for a week or two for one reason or another, I drop down both in distance and in speed when I return to the track. It takes a while to retune the motor, especially as you grow older and more especially if you are running with a scarred heart.

Andy was in exceptionally good condition and he had made reservations for the two of us at the Sheraton Boston a couple of months before. So I had a place to stay and someone to lend me moral support if I wanted to appear as an unofficial—and unwelcome—participant.

By the second week in April, I had run seven miles with no ill effects and I figured that, if I could go that far in the marathon, it would be worth the trip to Boston. I told my wife that I was going and she said that she thought I had lost my mind. But she had recovered from her first fear that I was going to drop dead if I climbed a flight of stairs, so she did not object too seriously.

I didn't tell Jerry. There seemed to be no point in doing that, and I didn't want to argue with him.

I stayed on the same schedule of running, usually five miles a day, one day a week more, sometimes up to nine, and my heart thumped along on its rather erratic way as dependably as the motor in a Model A Ford. Not ready for the Indianapolis 500 by any stretch of the imagination, but useful and dependable.

Once you have survived a crisis of one kind or another, a kind of euphoria sets in and I suppose that is what happened to me during the few weeks left before the marathon. After I had recovered from the shock and gotten over my excessive awareness of my heart, I ran as easily and as happily as I had ever done.

I suppose if I had never read the report, I might have run more and better, possibly with no ill effect. The report slowed me down quite a lot, and maybe that was a good thing, but I don't know now and I certainly didn't know in the days before the marathon.

The marathon became a kind of a symbol for me, I think. If I could run in it without dropping out in the first half mile, it would prove to me, at least, that my heart was stronger than the Cornell Medical Research doctors thought it was. I made up my mind that I would not run beyond any discomfort, or even beyond the slight chest pains I had felt when I first began running.

During this time, I tried to find some evidence from other post-cardiac patients who had run distances, but I could not find anything to support either my idea, that long runs are good, or evidence that long runs were fatal.

I guess it took a long time for the medical profession to get over the idea that a post-cardiac patient should spend the rest of his life as a semi-invalid. If I live long enough to prove my own theory that the damaged heart thrives on long, slow exercise, it may take years for that idea to be accepted.

I hope I live to see it.

Chapter Eighteen /

There must be hundreds of marathons run in the United States in the course of a year, but for some reason no other has ever achieved the publicity of the Boston Marathon, run from Hopkinton, Massachusetts, to the Prudential Building in downtown Boston every year on Patriot's Day, in late April.

In spite of my deep interest in running, the Boston Athletic Association Marathon run Monday, April 19, 1971, was the first I had ever seen and the first certainly that I had ever run in.

Andy and I flew to Boston Sunday evening, leaving the airport about five and arriving in Boston an hour later, after the usual air traffic delays. The Sheraton Boston, where we stayed, was full of marathon runners and we met more on the street when we went out for dinner.

Marathon runners are not difficult to recognize; they are almost completely devoid of fat, so that even the skin on their faces is stretched paper thin. They are without heavy muscles, even in their legs. I saw only one heavily muscled runner in the more than eight hundred who showed up in Hopkinton on the morning of the race, and he finished well back.

Andy and I had breakfast early that morning; he had an enormous stack of hotcakes with melted butter and syrup, orange juice, cereal, toast, and tea. I settled for scrambled eggs, sausage, toast, and coffee. Although I knew I was not going to go the whole distance and that I was not even an official entrant, I could feel the first faint tingle of nerves in my stomach, much the same as I used to feel at school on the morning of a football game.

We dressed at the hotel; Andy looked rather disreputable in an old red sweat shirt and blue warm-up pants over his running gear, but I had the blue nylon sweat suit and red running shoes, which made me look much more of a runner than I am. We had chartered a cab, through the hotel, to take us to Hopkinton, some twenty-six miles away, and stopped on the way to pick up a hitchhiker in running gear, a youngster who had come from Philadelphia to run in the marathon for the first time.

He was even more nervous than I was, and with more cause, since he was hoping to finish in something less than three hours. Our cab went along part of the course for a while and Andy shook his head dolefully.

"I hate going out the way we'll be coming in for the race," he said. "It always seems so damned far. Maybe because it *is* so damned far."

The youngster, who was about twenty, smiled weakly; so did I. I had been thinking that it was not only a long way, but that there seemed to be more and bigger hills than I had thought the Boston area contained.

When we finally arrived in Hopkinton, it was about eleven in the morning and we went directly to the Hopkinton High School gym, where Andy got his official numbers to pin on the front and back of his running suit. The small gym was crowded with runners of a surprising variety of ages, from fourteen-year-olds to men in their sixties. Andy seemed to know most of them.

Dr. George A. Sheehan, the New Jersey cardiologist, was rubbing his legs with vaseline, seated on a small row of bleacher seats at one side of the gym. Dr. Sheehan, quoted earlier in this book on the benefits of running for heart patients, runs in the marathon each year.

Each official entrant in the marathon must present a doctor's certificate showing that he is physically fit to compete, then undergo a brief examination before running.

I had met Dr. Sheehan the night before, and he nodded and smiled.

"How do you feel?" he asked.

"Pretty good," I said. "What do you think you'll make it in?"

"I'd like to get under three hours," he said. "I've come close, but I haven't broken three hours yet." Dr. Sheehan is fifty-two years old, a medium-sized, compact man with the strong, wiry legs of a distance runner.

A tall, thin man who looked to be in his middle forties came up to him, looking worried.

"My blood pressure was up a little," he said. "What should I do about that, George?"

"Run and bring it down again," Sheehan said, grinning. He nodded doubtfully and walked away.

"He's all right," George said. "Probably a little nervous, just like all of us. He'll get over it in a mile or so."

Hal Higdon, a free-lance writer who has done a book on jogging, said hello to Andy and invited us to come to his hotel suite after the race. He looked gaunt and very fit, which indeed he is; he has finished the marathon consistently in under three hours and he ran this one in two hours, forty-three minutes and fifty-six seconds, which was good enough to place him ninety-fourth in a field of nearly nine hundred official entrants.

Erich Segal, the novelist who wrote the best seller *Love Story*, was in the gym, attracting no great attention. He has run in fifteen of the last sixteen marathons here, but debated about this one for some time since the instant fame which came his way after the overwhelming success of his book interrupted his training.

Trying to explain what prompted him to run again, Segal, in an interview the day before the race, had said, "Call it humanism. Call it health. Call it folly." Call it whatever, it had brought Segal back, a thin man with long, bushy hair and a strained expression. He finished, too, but in somewhat slower time than he is used to, probably a result of too many literary lunches.

"I think I should have had one more day's rest," Sheehan says now. "It's hard to know when you are your own coach. I debated with myself Friday on whether or not to run, then did a slow five, but maybe I should have rested. I know Bill Bowerman sometimes gives his Oregon track team three days off before a big meet."

"Well, it's too late to do anything about it now," Andy said, cheerfully. He was trying to pin the numbers on his singlet, with no success because his hands were shaking. I finally took the running shirt and the numbers from him and pinned them on.

"I always get this way," Andy said ruefully. "I guess it's the old adrenalin."

"What did you have for breakfast?" I asked Dr. Sheehan.

"French toast with syrup, an English muffin with jelly, and a cup of coffee," he said. "Lots of sugar."

The night before, most of the joggers in the restaurant where Andy and I had eaten filled up on spaghetti. Contrary to the widely held belief among football players that a pregame steak provides the most strength, distance runners opt for the energy provided by carbohydrates.

Only one runner, a burly Canadian in his thirties, had eaten roast beef; after dinner, he had a strawberry sundae and several other runners immediately ordered the same thing. I asked Andy about it later and he grinned.

"That's Lauren Buck," he said. "He ran about two thirty-five last year, so a lot of guys figure the same diet might get them in under three, but it won't."

By now Andy had put on his shirt, with the numbers pinned on slightly askew, and we walked out of the gym into the bright, rather brisk morning. On the grass outside, runners were loping back and forth easily, warming up; I decided to save my energy and warm up during the first two or three miles of the race.

Andy and I walked through the crowd to the road and down the road to the starting point, exactly twenty-six miles 385 yards from the Prudential Building in Boston where the race would end. It was about a quarter to twelve and the little road was jammed with runners crowded close together to get as near the starting line as possible. A few minutes later, the fifty or sixty really serious competitors were installed at the head of the mob, where they could get away to a fast start without having to run over the main body of runners.

I found our cab driver at the side of the road and told him to wait until the field had been gone for forty-five minutes or so, then to follow along slowly.

"I don't know how far I'm going," I said. "But it certainly won't be all the way. After about five miles, start looking along the side of the road for me. I'll be leaning against a tree."

"You'll make it," he said.

"Look for me anyway," I told him.

I crowded back into the pack next to Andy and looked at my watch. It was nearly twelve and the runners were restless, some of them jogging in place and shaking their arms. Andy stood quietly enough and Dr. Sheehan looked placid and relaxed. I suddenly wished whole-heartedly that I had been able to keep in good training steadily, so that I could enter with some hope of finishing.

I thought fleetingly that I would run until I dropped and then realized how stupid that would be. I decided I would go until I was pleasantly tired, then stop and wait for the taxi.

Then the gun went off and for the first few hundred yards, while the huge pack of runners sorted itself out, no one could go very fast, so I felt inconspicuous enough. There were a few other runners in sweat suits and without numbers, I had noticed earlier.

There were also a few women, also without numbers

since the Boston Athletic Association does not allow women to compete officially. That will be changed for the 1972 marathon, since more and more women run in the race anyway and quite a few of them finish.

The first half mile or so of the marathon is downhill, for the most part. You go down the road to the town square of Hopkinton, turn right and run down a long gentle slope, past trees and houses, with people on both sides of the road. Most of them have papers with a list of the runners' names and numbers so that they can shout encouragement to the runners they know or have heard about. Most of them shouted compliments to Segal, who said after the race that his arms were nearly as tired from waving as his legs were from running.

Since I didn't have a number, no one said anything to me. I went along very slowly, dropping back as the race went along, but not worrying about it since I had no compulsion to stay among the front runners. I wanted to stay comfortably in the middle of the pack and I did for a mile or so, until the course began to climb a hill.

I went up the hill even more slowly and felt myself begin to sweat, a good sign usually because it means I have warmed up and the running will become easier. The only difficulty I was having at this time was with my sweat pants. I had stowed my stopwatch and valuables in the pockets and the jogging dragged them lower and lower on my hips so that about every hundred yards or so I had to hitch up my pants.

I considered stopping and taking them off but decided that it wasn't worth the trouble.

I reached the top of the small hill thankfully and went down, trying to resist the temptation to speed up. Most of the runners were ahead of me by now and I reflected that all of them, to be eligible, had run a marathon in under four hours and I hadn't run a marathon at all. I felt pretty good; I suppose I had gone about two miles and there were still a few runners behind me. I looked over my shoulder at them and at the motorcycle police behind them, holding back the stream of cars trailing the field.

In the next couple of miles, the field strung out so that most of the runners were on the shoulder of the road and the cars could pass. Along the side of the road, bystanders offered oranges and drinks and some of the runners took them, but I felt it would be unfair for me to, since I wasn't going all the way.

I came to another long hill and began to toil up it, my legs feeling tired, and a young woman trotted by me, followed by a boy who looked to me to be about ten years old. Neither of them seemed to be in any distress, but the hill, which must have been a mile long, was sapping my legs.

I reached the top and figured I had run four or five miles and decided I would go to the bottom and decide there how much farther to run. I looked behind me and there were a few stragglers toiling along, but the motorcycles were not far away.

By the time I reached the bottom and started up, they were on my heels. My legs were tired, but my breathing was all right, so I went on for another half mile or so, then began looking for a deserted spot beside the road where I could stop and wait for the taxi.

I finally found one and slowed down and walked a while, then stopped and hitched up my pants and leaned against a tree. The cars with the people following the race began to come by and someone hollered, "The finish line is in Boston!" I waved and yelled, "Cramp!" and pointed to the calf of my right leg.

More cars came by and often enough the passengers shouted insults at me of one kind or another, but I replied, "Cramp!" each time and began to wonder if my cab driver had gotten lost. There are buses, called meat wagons, which trail the marathon field to pick up dropouts with legitimate cramps or blisters or whatever, but they wouldn't start sweeping up the debris quite so soon.

Finally, the cab pulled up and I got in. The driver, a rather elderly Italian man, looked at me disappointedly and shook his head.

"You din' go very far," he said sadly.

"Far enough," I said. "How many miles was it?"

"I don' know," he said, shrugging. "I din' check my speedometer."

I figured out later that I had run about five miles, not a very strong performance, but, under the circumstances, about as well as I expected to do. I could very probably have gone another two or three miles, but I was anxious to get back to Boston and watch the finish of the race.

By the time we had reached the hotel and I had showered and changed, it was only about thirty minutes before the leading runners were due to show up at the top of the sloping street leading down to the finish line at the Prudential Building. I walked over from the hotel to watch.

The streets were packed with spectators and I stood among them, looking up at the corner where the first runner would appear. It was a good-natured, enthusiastic crowd; many of them had portable radios so that they knew who the leaders were.

The day had turned hot and windy and the time was not going to be a record, but when the first runner made the turn and started the two-hundred-yard dash for the tape, the crowd broke into cheers, as enthusiastically as if they were watching a world record performance.

The first runner was a surprise. He was a dark, gaunt man with a long, loping stride, a thick mustache, and salt etching white lines on his drawn face. He was followed closely by a smaller runner, who dropped back quickly as the winner spurted for the tape.

The winner, a dark **hor**se, was Señor Alvaro Mejia, a Colombian, thirty years old and unemployed. The second-place finisher was the favorite, Pat McMahon from Ireland, a considerably younger man.

The time was two hours, eighteen minutes and forty-five seconds, which is not bad for a thirty-year-old.

Chapter Nineteen /

I waited for Andy to finish as the crowd slowly thinned out and runner after runner made the turn at the top of the hill and finished the final two hundred yards. Some of them staggered, some shuffled, and a few, in a strange, desperate last effort to move up a notch in the order of finish, managed a sprint. Sometimes two runners sprinted together in a personal duel.

Andy finally made the turn a little more than an hour after the winner, running slowly and painfully, his face a bright red from the sun, obviously not far from exhaustion. I watched him shamble by the finish line, then followed him into the basement of the Prudential Building, transformed into an impromptu locker room and first-aid station.

The floor was covered with worn distance runners, lying about in various states of shock. As I wandered around looking for Andy, I was surprised to see just how much the race had taken out of the runners; some of them looked like basket cases, their faces grimy and sweat-streaked, the feet blistered, and the most common expression was one of pain.

I found Andy lying on the floor with his feet in the air.

"That's it," he said. "My God, that's it. Never again, do you hear me, never again."

"You look like death warmed over," I said to him kindly. "Can I get you anything?"

"A drink," he said. "Gatorade. Anything."

I brought him two glasses of Gatorade and he gulped them down and shuddered.

"My legs are killing me," he said. "And I've got blisters all over my feet. I don't know why I do this. I must be insane."

I looked around the basement, which had taken on the appearance of an emergency field hospital after a major attack, and shook my head.

"You must be," I said. "You ran about three thirty-one or -two, as near as I could judge by my wrist watch."

"It was tough," Andy said. "Too much wind. And I took the first ten miles too fast. I tried to stay with Sheehan and a couple of his friends and I knew I shouldn't be doing it but I was too stupid to slow down."

After he had rested for a half hour, I helped him back to the hotel, only about a hundred yards away. He hobbled along painfully, barely able to climb the stairs out of the basement.

"I'll be all right," he said when he reached the elevators to his room. "I'll soak in a tub for about an hour and I'll feel fine. Then I want a few beers."

"I'll buy," I told him. "You have earned them."

While I waited for Andy in the bar, I talked to some of the runners who had finished ahead of him and who had already recuperated enough to have a few beers and rehash the race for the first of the hundreds of times it would be gone over in the next few hours.

Most distance runners are introspective and articulate, since they participate in a lonely sport which gives them a great deal of time to think. The most articulate may be Dr. Sheehan, who told me how he had felt during the run, then wrote about it very well in a column he contributes to his local newspaper.

After going over his preparation for the marathon, he details the day of the race:

Monday 7:30 A.M.: Up for breakfast and Boylston Street is already alive. Some guys are, mirabile dictu, already warming up; others waiting for the 8:30 bus. We have arranged for a ride out so breakfast is leisurely. French toast covered with syrup, an extra English muffin with jelly and a cup of coffee. I fill my muscles with sugar while reading Erich Segal in the *Times* . . . the Yale prof who has been running the Boston since 1955.

10:30 A.M.: The Hopkinton gym is madness. One thousand runners plus friends, officials, newsmen, and a movie crew doing a documentary. Only problems left are what to wear and the pace. The weather, cold in Boston, is warm here and still changing. Start with a long-sleeved turt-leneck shirt and my light Jasper running shirt (it will be Boston College before the crowd knows what a Jasper is). I pop outside for a minute and come back in. Discard the Jasper shirt and rip the sleeves off the turtleneck. Back outside. Still too much. Transfer the numbers to the Jasper shirt, and I'm down to my summer garb. One last thought. Put on my gloves and ear band. The ultimate schizophrenic outfit.

11:58 A.M.: On the line with Bob Milner, the thirty-four-year-old Colgate coach and compan-ion for the entire route last year in 3:02. This year, says Bob, we will break three and he has the wrist watch and checkpoints (pinned to his shirt) to prove it. Well, I am not getting any younger. May as well go for broke. It's noon, and we're on our way.

1:07 P.M.: We hit Cemetery Street in Natick, the ten-mile mark, five minutes ahead of last year but I'm already sweating and hurting. Gloves and ear bands discarded. Covered with Gatorade poured over the head. Too soon to take liquids.

1:40 P.M.: The pace is telling. It has already tolled for Bob Milner who is suddenly unable to keep up. I am left without watch, checkpoints, companion, confidence. Into the hills now and wondering what I have left. Heartbreak, the last hill, will tell. I have passed the two girls and some others I have never beaten and this could be my day. But Heartbreak says no. I am reduced to a crawling, grotesque walk-run before the summit.

There's nothing left now but misery. The down-hill from Boston College is torture.

2:48 P.M.: Still two miles to go when I see the time on a bank. The three-hour marathon must wait another year. But I'm going to finish. For the first time I'm certain of that. Even with the new pain. The blisters are here. The last 200 yards are impossible. Use as few muscles as possible and keep moving. You are an awkward, musclebound, barely moving, dimly aware human being with just one idea. Reach those people at the finish line. Then the finish and the pain stops and the joy starts and you are sitting with your feet in the fountain and everybody is talking and it's over for another year.

Since most distance runners are neither doctors nor prose stylists, I doubt that anyone will match Dr. Shee-han's crisp and moving account of what it feels like to run in the marathon for a long time.

For Segal, the novelist and professor, the marathon is a more mystical experience.

"I'm sick of the limelight," Segal said to a ring of writers after the race, swigging Gatorade glass after glass as he talked. His thin, intense face framed in unruly wiry hair, which kept falling in his eyes, he seemed very in-tent upon making his point.

"This was the toughest marathon I have run in," he said. "And I have run in fifteen out of the last sixteen, starting when I was in school. But this was the best, too. It was the best because of what I've been through this last year. Fame and all the pressures that go with it."

He swiped ineffectually at his hair and gulped down a glass of the Gatorade.

"I don't mind what the critics have said about my work," he went on. "That's their job and their right. But the personal attacks, the speculations on my upbringing, the talk about my background. That hurt."

(During the race, Crichton ran with Segal for a while. "I saw a good piece about you in the paper the other day," he said to make conversation. "It must be the only one anyone has written about me for a long time," Segal replied.)

"I'll tell you why this has been the best marathon for me," Segal went on in the basement of the Prudential Building. "Because it was a letdown for all the people who say—or think—I have changed and gotten too big to run in the marathon."

He looked as defiant as a small, thin man with too much hair, worn by fatigue, can look.

"They didn't think I would ever run again," he said. "They said Segal is too busy sipping champagne from girls' slippers." He grinned and brandished his paper cup of Gatorade.

"You can tell them for me that I sip Gatorade from girls' track shoes," he said.

By the time Crichton had soaked away his aches and come down to the bar for his first cold draft beer, he had already decided to run again in the 1972 marathon.

"It was too windy out there today," he said. "I can do better than that. I know it. How far did you go?"

I told him and he laughed.

"You got one consolation," he said.

"What's that?"

"You finished first," he said and laughed immoderately. I think that on weaker types the long strain of the marathon brings on a touch of hysteria.

After Crichton had had several more imported beers at my expense, we walked over to the Hotel Lennox, where Higdon was holding open house in his suite, serving cold beer instead of cocktails. The two-room suite was crowded and most of the runners were discussing the difficulties of the afternoon run. Only Crichton seemed crippled by it.

In the hall outside the suite were stacks of running equipment—windbreakers, shorts, running shirts, shoes, and a stack of Hal's books. Business seemed brisk; runners and joggers are like most hobbyists in that they have an insatiable desire for more and more modern equipment, although it is doubtful that a new pair of shoes ever took thirty minutes off anyone's time for the marathon.

After we had been there for over an hour, a rather elderly, heavyset gentleman arrived, still in his running gear and sweating profusely. I thought at first that he must have gone out for a post-marathon jog, which seemed a very unlikely event.

He was drinking Gatorade thirstily when I approached him and introduced myself. He smiled and shook my hand vigorously.

"Came all the way from New Mexico for this," he said. "I wouldn't miss it for the world."

"Did you run in the marathon?" I asked, thinking he might have been a spectator who went out for a run of his own when it ended.

"Oh, yes," he said. "That's what I came for."

"Did you finish?" I asked him, thinking I might find at least one man who had not done any better than I had. He wore a hand-lettered number on his sweat-drenched running shirt, so I knew that he was not an official entrant.

"Of course," he said.

"What was your time?"

"I just finished," he said, surprised. "Came right over here from the finish line. Didn't even stop to shower." That, of course, was apparent.

"Cramps slow you up?" I asked, expecting him to use my own excuse.

"Not a bit," he said. "I finished in six hours and forty-five minutes. That's my best time ever. Last year it took me seven and a half hours."

I discovered later that he was in his late sixties. I suppose if he lives long enough (and he looks as strong as an ox), he may get in under four hours.

The party broke up fairly early and Andy and I and three other runners had dinner at the Beachcomber Restaurant in the hotel, where I watched in disbelief as they put away enormous helpings of ribs, chicken, rice, grog, and desserts. Certainly the marathon develops an enormous appetite.

I listened during dinner as they went over the race again, damn nearly step by step. It was interesting up to a point—about five miles from the starting line, where I had given up to wait for my cab driver.

It did not last long. A big meal, grog, and a twenty-six-mile run combine to make even the hardiest of marathon runners a bit sleepy. I hadn't run twenty-six miles, but I made up for it with the grog.

As Andy limped along beside me to the elevator, I looked at him curiously. His face was drawn and walking was clearly very painful.

"You figure it's worth it?" I asked him.

"Worth it!" he said, waking up an elderly bellhop. Andrew has a voice which I suppose could best be described as penetrating. When he is making a point, it is earsplitting. Now it was earsplitting.

"I wouldn't miss it for the world!" he went on, leaning against the wall while we waited for the elevator. "Didn't you have fun?"

"Sure," I said, helping him into the elevator. "*I* had fun. You damned near killed yourself. Remember what you said right after the race?"

"I say that every year," Andy said. "So does everyone else. But we get over it."

I tried to read for a while when I got to bed, but I could not concentrate. I went over the day in my mind, from the start through the disaster area of the locker room in the Prudential Building.

From the rather modest program of jogging that I had followed for over two years, I knew how much time and energy and sweat had gone into preparing the eight hundred-odd runners who had finished the marathon that afternoon. In terms of time and miles, it was staggering.

For by far the majority of them, the race offered no glory, no fame, not even recognition in their hometown papers. They ran for the pure pleasure of running. Or, to be more accurate, the pure pleasure of having run.

I remembered what Andy had said to me a couple of years before.

"There aren't a hell of a lot of things you can do in the

world which give you a really solid sense of accomplishment," he said. "I mean a feeling that you have done something well and that you have done it at some cost in effort and application that requires determination beyond what most people have or are willing to use. Finishing the marathon is one thing that you have to have devoted a lot of hours and a lot of determination and a lot of pain to doing. It makes you feel good to have done it."

"That's good for one time," I said. "I can understand that. But why do it over and over. You're never going to win the marathon."

"It gets to be a habit," he said. "I mean, after you have run long enough, you can't really stop running. You get addicted."

"I see," I had said then, although I didn't see.

We walked slowly down the hall to our adjoining rooms and said good night, and it wasn't until later, when I remembered what Andy had said two years before, that I realized what the marathon runners reminded me of.

They were all addicts.

Chapter Twenty /

Andrew, to put it mildly, is not one of the great admirers of the Wright brothers. When we went to Boston, he bought a one-way ticket on the plane, hoping that he could hitchhike a ride back by car. No one offered him a ride, so he had to fly back with me.

We were supposed to get an early plane, but he slept late, used up a good deal more time trying to find a ride, then packed very slowly, hoping we would miss the plane. But we didn't, so we flew back to New York.

It was a quick flight and a reasonably pleasant one until we landed. Andy controlled his fears reasonably well; sometimes he sounded almost normal when he talked, although he did not make much sense.

We landed at La Guardia, the plane coming in fast.

When the pilot put on the brakes, there was a muffled explosion, the plane leaned sharply to the left and veered to the side of the runway before the pilot straightened it out again. It was still leaning to the left as he brought it to a stop.

"God Almighty!" Andy said. "What was that!"

"Sounded like a blow out," I said. "We're home and dry now."

"I damn near had a heart attack!" Andy said.

"That's funny," I said. "I didn't."

It has been a while since the marathon as I write this. I am still jogging and I'm still alive and, hopefully, I'll still be alive when you read this. If I'm not, you must have waited for the paperback edition, because the publisher, in signing the contract for this book, made it a rather unusual one.

Normally, I get half the advance when I sign the contract for a book, the other half when I submit an acceptable manuscript.

This time, it was one third on signing, one third on completion of the manuscript, and one third on publication. So if I died of a heart attack between finishing the book and its publication, the publisher would be off the hook for at least one third of the advance.

I don't blame the publisher and I signed the contract willingly. I suppose, if the editors had had the opportunity to read the Cornell Medical Research report on me, they might have insisted that the advance be withheld in its entirety until publication.

I have had a little more time to evaluate the experience of the last two and a half years and I have thrown away the stopwatch and I run now for pleasure, as well as to give my heart and lungs enough exercise to keep them fit.

Certainly the last thing I would do is to recommend to other post-cardiac patients the program that I have survived. Occasionally I meet another heart-attack victim on the track and almost invariably he is shocked to find out how far I'm running.

There are, of course, quite a few post-cardiac joggers; the West Side YMCA has a closely supervised program for heart patients, based on jogging, with some thirty runners, and there are other such programs in Ys throughout the country. Since my work schedule is erratic and since I travel extensively, it is impossible for me to take part in such a program, so that I have worked out my own program. I began going fairly long distances more or less by accident, primarily because I felt no ill effects from running and because my endurance built up rather easily.

There are heart conditions that preclude running entirely. Mine did not happen to be one and I don't think it is one now. But only time will tell that. At any rate, I feel better running and taking vitamin E and I still smoke and drink and, at the moment, I'm still alive.

That's all anyone reading this sentence can say.

I have, more or less, given up any ambition to run in the marathon. After looking over the wreckage in the basement of the Prudential Building in Boston after the marathon of 1971, I doubt that my heart, at its sturdiest, could have taken that kind of punishment.

But, if you haven't had a heart attack and if you have trained yourself to the point where, like Andy and Dr. Sheehan and Erich Segal and all the rest of the 800 addicts who ran in the marathon and finished, the odds are pretty strongly in your favor.

I would like to run again in the marathon, however, with a goal somewhat less ambitious than finishing, even finishing like my old friend from New Mexico, showing up at Hal Higdon's party still sweating from nearly seven hours on the road, at least two of them all alone and stared at by curious, and sometimes unfriendly, dogs and children.

I think Dr. Sheehan's story of his run in 1971 pointed up a reasonable goal for me. "1:07 P.M.: We hit Cemetery Street in Natick, the ten-mile mark, five minutes ahead of last year, but I'm already sweating and hurting. . . ."

In my next marathon, I would like to make it all the way to Cemetery Street.

If I don't get there before.